"Within a healthy body any diseased organ can be healed with the help of cupping or leeching." — *Avicenna*

"It's impossible to enumerate all the diseases that can be treated by leech therapy…and, oftentimes, leeches prevent people from having surgeries, especially in cases such as hemorrhoids, varicose veins, or blood clots."
— *Dr. Svetlana Comissarov*

"This living pill carries a whole pharmacy within itself! And when it attaches to the skin, it infuses our blood with more than a hundred different biologically active substances."
— *Dr. Vladimir Kozirev*

"After undergoing a bypass surgery, many people are destined to take pills for years. The chemicals in them damage the stomach lining, the liver and the quality of the blood. I have achieved incredible results with leech therapy, which dissolves small clots while not having any negative impact on other organs." — *Dr. Vladimir Koklushenkov, family doctor*

"I have known many women who were unable to conceive for a long time; but after a leech therapy session they didn't have any problems getting pregnant." — *Dr. Vladimir Kozirev*

"When a new antibiotic comes along, so does a new disease. To break this vicious circle, more and more scientists and doctors are becoming convinced that it's time to resort to the natural ways of healing." — *Dr. Vladimir Koklushenkov, family doctor*

Leech Therapy

*An Introduction to a
Natural Healing Alternative*

By Matt Isaac

**Leech Therapy: An Introduction
to a Natural Healing Alternative**
By Matt Isaac

ISBN: 978-0-9836339-1-4

Published by Bread Line Publishing

Printed in the USA

Design & Layout by EditWriteDesign.com

Disclaimer: The purpose of this work is to provide as accurate information as possible regarding the subject of leech therapy. The actions and ideas put forth in this book are not intended to replace a consultation with a physician or other medical specialists. The author and/or publisher are not engaged in any professional medical services and are not liable for any injury, loss, or other damages purportedly caused by the use of the information found in this book. Do not attempt to apply any technique described in this book on your own, without first receiving proper training under the supervision of an expert.

Acknowledgement

For my Mother

Contents

5. Leech Therapy Process   27

6. Leeches in the Medical Practice   51

7. Step by Step Instructions   59

1

<u>Introduction</u>

The mission

We all get sick sometimes. And when we do, we frantically try to learn what we can do to make it stop—immediately. But when we are presented with the options to remedy our bad fortune, we seldom inquire about the cure's origin or ask questions about how it works and why it is the best approach for us. Meanwhile, the approach constantly changes and the new becomes the best while the old is quickly forgotten.

People around the world spend billions of dollars searching for something original, unusual, something totally new. But most of the time, we forget about the things already available to us. And certain truths that were discovered many years ago are still true today. The medical field is no exception. That is why I invite you to join me on a journey into the past to dig up some valuable knowledge about medicinal leeches, which were once popular medicine in Imperial Rome, Western Europe, ancient Eastern medicine, and Russia.

While currently thriving in a medical rebirth and being recognized by hundreds of doctors and published research in Russia, the medicinal leech has received very little support here in the United States. In Russia, a country that has had one of the richest histories and medical successes with this healing method, people have put forth a great deal of time and effort into researching and observing these unorthodox little healers.

I have compiled a great deal of information from the Russian literature, available today, that will introduce you to some fascinating facts about leeches and hirudotherapy (*leech therapy*), the methods that were employed during the past centuries, information about the uses of medicinal leeches today, and its valuable implications for modern medicine, in the hopes that one day leeches will receive their much-deserved recognition.

I wrote this book for people who are interested in learning more about leech therapy. It may be those who have had great success with leech therapy and want to learn how to safely and effectively administer it at home. Others might be suffering and looking for a method of healing that works after they have exhausted all other options. Or it could be a doctor with an open mind looking to expand his/her knowledge beyond what universities and medical schools had to offer. Or it may be a homeopathic healer looking to increase his/her healing arsenal. And even if you might be indifferent toward or skeptical of hirudotherapy at first, I hope this book will give you enough motivation and knowledge to trust a leech to help you on your journey to health. This path should enable you to gradually liberate yourself from relying on pills and doctors and to understand that health is a lifetime career that requires constant work, discipline, and attention.

Brief history

In the past, medical practice accepted leeches as the cure for almost any illness. They were especially popular in Western Europe at the end of the 18th century and in first half of 19th century. At one time, Russia alone used up to thirty million leeches a year for medical purposes. Perhaps the main reason why people still recognize leech therapy at all is because it was once the main arsenal of medical practice and was regarded as a natural path of reestablishing a person's health.

And perhaps the most monumental work written about leech therapy was produced in 1859, St. Petersburg, Russia. This work, entitled "The study of medicinal leeches," was completed only because the author, Voskresensky, was instructed to do so by the medical department of the Russian Military. The book documented the history of leeches in Russia and abroad, as well as their practical uses for human benefit. Voskresensky also noted that in no other country, except in Russia, did leeches play such an important economic and medical role.

During the second half of 19th century, however, the favorable attitude towards leeches quickly deteriorated when it became popular opinion that these little creatures caused infection. As a result, doctors started to believe that it was easier and healthier to conduct bloodletting through surgical means by making small incisions in the veins, rather than using leeches.

By the beginning of the 20th century, leeches almost completely disappeared from the medical practice and were quickly removed from standard medicine and placed into the homeopathic category. Soon, the leech had found itself moved from the reference section of a bookstore and placed into the comic section instead. This quick demise of leech therapy can also be attributed to the fact that, as technology and science progressed, nobody took the time and effort to learn more about the medicinal properties of leeches.

Leech therapy today

For many years, leech therapy was regarded as a cure-all, only to be later mocked and thrown into oblivion. Today, people mostly use the pharmaceutical approach to healing rather than choosing leech therapy, even though it has been proven to be safe and without side effects. But, sometimes, it pays to revert to the old and proven techniques and practices, rather than discover new ones, which may come with a higher price tag and even a larger margin of error.

Moreover, modern medicine has proven to be ineffective in so many different areas, adding yet another reason for a growing interest in leech therapy. To any reasonable person, especially a doctor, the mismatch between today's medical theory and its applications is painfully obvious. The general public is often treated to a handful of chemicals, instead of being offered a natural and safe path to healing (such as leech therapy). It is true that chemicals can offer a quick fix of symptoms, but for a lengthier and more involved treatment, with longer lasting results, many people are now beginning to turn to alternative healing methods.

Luckily, there are a number of different approaches to medicine. Although our current culture encourages one to seek health in the doctor's office (with a quick fix of a pill or a surgery), alternative medicine clinics frequently emphasize that people are responsible for their own health. And while this kind of therapy often goes against conventional wisdom, the more people learn about its benefits, the more they seek these alternative kinds of options. And recently many around the world have discovered leech therapy.

But even with this burgeoning comeback of the public interest in leech therapy, the experience accumulated in Russia (and other countries) is all but forgotten, and modern data regarding this type of therapy is scarce. Today, leech therapy is again in its infancy and still requires more work if we are to recover all the lost knowledge about this method of healing.

2

A Holistic Approach to Healing

Why leeches?

The leech is haunted by a terrible paradox. Leech therapy peaked in popularity a few centuries ago when there was little research or scientific facts available to back up its benefits. Today, however, when we do have proven facts and studies of the numerous advantages of using leech therapy, there are very few people who recognize this method, let alone actually apply it. But since many examples of the great and, at times, indispensable uses of leech therapy have been already documented, it would be unwise to continue to ignore it.

Leech treatments are simple, inexpensive, and can be conducted in hospitals, as an outpatient procedure, or at home. It can be used as a sole approach to healing, as well as in combination with other treatments. This type of therapy is indispensible when it comes to many chronic diseases and performs as good as, if not better than, some standard medical procedures, which may be more costly, have higher risks of complications, and are usually accompanied by a handful of drugs with nasty side effects.

If leeches are fresh, clean, and properly used, complications are virtually non-existent. And when the rare ones arise, they are not difficult to treat. This is especially important for people who are using leech therapy in household conditions.

In case of an illness that has severe symptoms, the effects of leech therapy are felt almost immediately. The patient experiences reduced pain, diminished swelling, and a drop in body temperature. Moreover, leech therapy can be used to reduce the duration of a disease, prevent possible complications, and support a good state of health.

Leech therapy can be used as an anti-atherosclerotic treatment (*atherosclerosis is when artery walls become thinker and harder due to buildup of cholesterol*); against muscle spasms and high blood pressure (*hypertension*); against thrombosis; and to fight many more other diseases. The list of leech therapy applications is so long, that it would lead you to believe that modern medicine would employ leeches as full time doctors. But, unfortunately, that is not the case. Instead, billions of dollars are poured into designing "quick fixes" for the masses.

Yet, the most important aspect of leech treatment is designing a strategy that is tailored specifically for the patient, for each will require individual results. This is indeed labor intensive and does not allow a doctor to plug in a cookie cutter answer, but proper planning will result in the best outcome and should eliminate any complications. Therefore, the specialist should always first consider the condition of the patient, the strength of the immune system, the condition of the organs closest to the area of attachment, their ability to function, and the patient's psychological readiness.

Recognizing troubles early

Today, most people suffer from some type of chronic illness (sometimes more than one), and almost everyone thinks of themselves as being sick in some form or another. But, sometimes, we have difficulty recognizing the progression of our diseases. Being able to carefully assess our overall health can lead us to simpler healing options and positive lifestyle changes.

Most illnesses don't just fall upon us all of a sudden. They develop gradually and in stages. And the earlier we see the signs, the better we can defend ourselves.

Stage 1: The first stage of the disease often occurs when no specific symptoms can be detected yet. It happens when all reserves of the immune system become depleted and its resistance to illness decreases. In many cases, these conditions manifest themselves through unusually strong reactions of the organism to mild physical strain, mental stress, or stimulation. So, while no disease can be identified yet and it is impossible to make any medical diagnosis, a skilled specialist should be able to recognize the situation and propose a program that includes the overall strengthening of the organism.

Stage 2: The second stage is recognized by detecting a few signs of the disease, or "micro-symptoms." If these symptoms are ignored—as they often are—then the disease may progress further, since the body already lost its ability to fight off the illness. At this stage, the best course of action is to take steps toward natural healing such as hydrotherapy, fasting, or exercising.

Stage 3: The third stage is the one we are all too familiar with. This is when the symptoms are fully present, and we can no longer ignore them, even if we wanted to.

The importance of healthy blood circulation

Different people have different weaknesses. It is usually the "weakest link" that breaks first as soon as the deterioration process begins. Some people experience heart problems and headaches, while others experience pain in their joints, kidneys, stomachs, etc.

The following lifestyle and diet choices can lead to poor blood circulation and venous stasis:

- Not enough aerobic activity
- Constant stress
- Weak abdominal muscles and diaphragm
- Consuming foods high in sugar, refined flour, and chemical additives

But it is not always our fault. Many people are simply genetically predisposed to blood stasis in various tissues. These people usually have weaker lymphatic systems which may cause liver and gall bladder inability to handle overloads on a regular basis and may result in limited capacity of the liver to filter out waste and toxins.

Over time, these factors add up and can result in a poor blood circulation that puts tremendous stress on the metabolism. This stressful overload can lead to the accumulation of waste that stays in the digestive system and results in an increased amount of toxins and poisons which negatively affect mucous membranes and microcirculation systems (*responsible for the process of transporting blood through the tissues — i.e. capillaries*). This condition of poor blood circulation does not allow the body's "self-cleaning" system to work as efficiently as it should. Hence, the lack of "self-cleaning" may be identified as the root cause of many diseases we see today.

When microbes enter a healthy organism, they are usually destroyed by its immune system. Yet, it can be easily infected when tissues become unable to cleanse themselves and accumulate waste, which deteriorates and weakens them. As a result, the organism is unable to battle with even the puniest outside invaders.

To make a full recovery from any illness, it is necessary to clean the tissues and restore their ability to drain unnecessary wastes. And that is when the medicinal leech comes to the rescue.

The whole body treatment

Leech therapy is not just a surface treatment. It is a complex process that should be regarded as a holistic treatment for the entire body rather than a mechanical bleeding in one spot that benefits only the local organ(s).

When some tissues are damaged or perform irregularly due to a disruption in microcirculation (*the process of transporting blood through the tissues*), the organism as a whole begins to suffer. This disruption of microcirculation has shown to be the underlying cause of many diseases. The important cellular exchanges of nutrition and waste disposal occur in the blood vessels responsible for microcirculation. Leech therapy impacts vascular and lymphatic systems and spurs a biochemical reaction that results in the strengthening of the organism, immune system, and increased resistance to pathogenic factors of internal and external environments. Consequently, it restores the body temperature, normalizes blood pressure, regulates sugar levels, and ultimately helps to re-establish overall health.

Therapy begins at the moment the leech bites through the skin and the biological substances from the leech enter into the bloodstream. Naturally, the immune system is immediately alerted and automatically raises the patient's natural defenses to fight the invaders. This reaction often occurs due to the skin irritation, pain, and blood loss. The substances released by the leech can also activate the human immune system. And due to this activation, pathogenic microorganisms in the blood of a person (certain types of staph infection, strep infection, spirochete infection, etc.) are not only weakened, but also destroyed by the white cells (*neutrophilic leukocytes*); therefore, this reaction enhances their ability to catch and digest microbes and parts of destroyed cells in the bloodstream.

Following a therapy session, these reactions may spur a false feeling of being sick. But it is a necessary part of therapy that will ultimately help a patient to achieve overall healing. Besides, the impact of the leech therapy will largely depend on the sensitivity of the individual organism and the amount of irritation it creates. It will directly correspond to the number of leeches concentrated in one area. Meanwhile, the intensity of the body's reaction to the therapy will vary with illness; and it is vital to closely monitor how the organism is reacting during the process.

Some diseases require highly intensive therapy, while others should be treated with much lower intensity. Keep in mind though, that a small number of leeches in an area does not create a skin irritation and, in some instances, may not lead to the desired outcome. And at times, the amount of blood that leaves the organism is too small and might not be enough to create a desired effect. During a heavy procedure that uses a high quantity of leeches, the results are often amplified by the amount of blood leaving the body, which may act as an anti-inflammatory process.

Noticeable swelling and infection can only be treated with a larger quantity of leeches, while a slight swelling or minor infection requires a smaller quantity of leeches. This holds true for all parts of the body including the breathing system, extremities, mid-section, reproductive organs, etc.

In addition, leeches have a well-known anti-clotting agent that helps against blood clotting, therefore lessening the occurrence of thrombosis (*a formation of a blood clot inside a blood vessel that obstructs the flow of blood through the circulatory system*) and/or bloody expectoration (*act of bringing up and spitting out*).

Medicinal leeches also have a spectrum of highly-active biological substances within its body that, even in small amounts, is able to get rid of microbes in the newly-acquired blood. In this manner, the blood inside a leech remains fresh and infection free. According to I.Shishkinoj, the ability to absorb microbes (*phagocytosis — process of a cell engulfing solid particles*) by the white cells in the human body is increased two to three times during leech therapy. This same process is observed inside the leech, where the consumed blood is not only rid of microbes by immune cells (*phygocytes*), but also by the symbiotic bacteria that lives in the digestive tract of the leech. These wonderful properties guarantee that it is impossible for a leech to transmit an infection from one person to another. In fact, counter to popular belief, leech therapy can actually enhance the human ability to fight infections.

Biologically-active substances produced by a leech have the ability to relieve vascular spasms, while raising amount of oxygen and nutrients in tissues, expanding the vessels, lowering the blood pressure in the arteries, and soothing the pain. Additional clinical studies have shown leech therapy to have the ability to help sclerosis patients by restoring and strengthening blood circulation in the arteries, tissues and the vein system. Leech therapy can also help the body to process fat, leading to healthier vascular walls and reduced blood viscosity.

Finally, leeches may promote purification of an organism from poisonous substances and may be able to treat some organs that cannot be reached by other means.

People often wonder if they should use medicinal leeches only to strengthen the organism and get it "back on track" or to treat any developed diseases. The answer is—both, because the medicinal leech therapy is equally effective as a healing method and as a prophylactic (*preventative*) treatment. Whether a patient's health has completely deteriorated due to the advanced stages of a disease, or a person is merely looking to take preventative steps to avoid illness, leech therapy can be a viable option.

> *Note: To avoid complications, do not administer leech therapy to patients whose immune system has been severely compromised.*

3

These Wonderful Little Creatures

Common types of leeches

Since ancient times healers knew about leeches and paid close attention to them. Therefore, people quickly learned about leeches, their life, how to care for them, and how to grow them in a controlled environment.

Although there are many practical uses for the medicinal leech, few of these are known to the public. Most people's basic knowledge does not extend beyond the fact that leeches produce hirudin (*an anti-coagulant, something that prevents blood from clotting*). Learning about physical and biological attributes of a leech should equip you with necessary knowledge so that you will be able to choose the right treatment while understanding exactly how to achieve success in alleviating pain and suffering (or curing the illness altogether).

There are about four hundred different kinds of leeches. The ones that are most commonly used for therapy have distinct properties. Medicinal leeches are usually dark-brown, brown, dark green, green, or red-brown. It is possible to encounter leeches of other colors, although less often. On its back, the medicinal leech has six stripes that vary in color: red, light-brown, yellow or black; however, in many instances, it is difficult to detect the stripes because they may appear as rows of red or yellow dots. The sides of a leech are normally green, with a hint of yellow or olive shade. The belly is often motley colored with yellow, dark green, with black, grey or brown spots.

Hirudo medicinalis – commonly known as the medicinal leech, is brownish-olive. Its back is covered with black spots and has six intertwining reddish-yellow stripes. It has a bright belly. The medicinal leech's body is comprised of rings with a coarse surface. It has ten small eyes (five pairs) located near the front sucker. Both ends of the body are equipped with muscular suckers. A mouth is located on their front extremity, and a rectum is on the back end. The leech uses both ends of its body to stick to other objects. One of the largest populations of this kind of leech has been found in Ukraine. *Hirudo medicinalis* is considered the most effective leech used in the medical practice.

Hirudo officinalis – is dark green with six back stripes, but without spots. Its belly has a solid yellow color, and the rings around the body are smooth. It is sometimes referred to as the Hungarian leech, because of its origin. Today, it dwells mostly in Moldova, Krasnodar territory, and Armenia.

Hirudo Orientales – is much brighter than the other leeches. Along the back, it has narrow orange stripes covered with equally-spaced quadrilateral spots. The belly is black with green spots, which are equally-spaced as well.

Leeches unusable for medicinal use share the following characteristics:

- One color
- No stripes
- Hairy
- Very round dull heads

Both the medicinal and non-medicinal leeches may often have the same size and somewhat similar shape. Non-medicinal leeches, however, do not have the same advanced jaw structure, and their teeth are much duller. This means that a non-medicinal leech will oftentimes attach to the skin, but it will not have the ability to penetrate through it.

There are two varieties of non-medicinal leeches that are often mistaken for their medicinal cousins. The first is *Hoemopis vorax, Sawigni,* which has a smooth back with a muddy green color, dark belly, yellow sides and reddish-brown stripes. It excretes a lot of slime.

The second, *Aulocostamani grescens,* is a greenish-black creature with a yellow belly. It resides near freshwater. This kind can quickly attach to the skin of a swimming person or a drinking animal and deeply penetrate through the skin, potentially causing very serious bleeding with potentially lethal outcomes. One needs to be very cautious around these types.

Structure of the organism

The leech has a quite complex body structure. The largest part of a leech is the stomach and muscles, which make up about sixty-five percent of its organism. The body of the leech is not smooth; instead it is evenly cross-sectioned by a series of grooves and rings. The surface is covered by tiny suctions, which, at times, protrude from the body.

The head of a leech is pointy and is much narrower than the tail end. Leech's eyes are located on its upper lip, but they are almost unnoticeable. The triangular-shaped front suction opening consists of several layers that are designed to create a vacuum effect. A leech has three jaws—one horizontal and the other two lateral—all of which are equipped with pointy, sharp, little teeth. It is this efficient mechanism that allows the leech to bite through the skin, other soft tissues, or mucous membranes. These three internal jaws have up to sixty teeth that are used to bite through the skin and are shaped like semicircular saws.

The digestive system is located right behind the jaws, where it turns into the digestive track that makes up to two-thirds of the length of the leech's body. The stomach is made up of a series of tightly closed pouches that lead to the rectum. The tail end of the leech is much thicker and ends in a spherical suction on the belly. (Hint: When trying to differentiate the front from the tail end, it is helpful to look for the suction cup on the back end since it is larger and always visible.)

The length of an adult leech ranges from from two to four inches. The size of a leech, however, cannot serve as a definite criterion of its age. The average weight of a leech is about one-tenth of an ounce (2.5 grams). Record-sized leeches include a specimen with a length of seventeen and a half inches, a weight of thirty-nine grams, and a one-fifth inch rear sucker.

Artificial cultivation of leeches has revealed some very fascinating facts:

- Although leeches are able to go without feeding for several months at a time, they do not require fasting and are able to feed repeatedly without taking long breaks.
- Even with frequent feeding, they consume a great amount of blood with each meal.
- Their mass increases when they eat more frequently.
- With a regular meal schedule, medicinal leeches are able to survive and remain healthy for long periods of time.

Reproduction

The reproductive features of leeches are rather remarkable. They are hermaphrodites, meaning that leeches have both male and female organs. This rather complex reproductive structure is located on the center of the leech's belly, with the male organ being closer to the front sucker than the female one.

But leeches do not impregnate themselves. They usually mate with another leech, or sometimes two. This process can last from fifteen to eighteen minutes, and in the end, all participants can be left pregnant.

In nature, leeches usually mate in their third year of life. In artificial conditions, however, they may become ready to mate just after twenty-two months. For the most part, they will mate during spring, summer, and (at times) near the end of fall. Each mating period takes from thirty to forty days. After that, a leech makes a cocoon filled with a protein-like substance and eggs. The cocoon is similar to that of a silkworm and contains anywhere from fifteen to thirty eggs. Leeches bury these cocoons in the ground along the edges of the shores of their habitat, preferably between stones.

In favorable conditions, especially in sunny weather, newborns hatch in forty days and crawl out of the small opening on the tip of the cocoon. They are so small that they can be detected only when they move. Despite their small size, they have large appetites following hatching, and they act very similar to their parents by getting their nutrition (blood) from frogs and tadpoles.

A leech develops very slowly, especially in the first two years. It can take five to eight years for a leech to fully mature; and it may live up to twenty years. Under natural conditions, leeches reach a necessary size for therapy no earlier than in five years, although they may still be used for medical purposes in their third and fourth year. In an artificial environment, a leech can be grown to the necessary weight for medicinal use—1.5 to 2.0 grams—in twelve to thirty-six months. But its lifespan is much shorter—three to four years on average; although some may live up to eight years.

Environment and survival

Medical leeches live in freshwater reservoirs: ponds, lakes, and small rivers. Leeches breathe through their skin, absorbing the oxygen in the water. They love fresh flowing water, but not wells. Water, however, is not their only habitat for they can live in wet grounds, clay, and moss by burying themselves deep into their chosen home. Once there, they can remain dormant for months. But wherever they reside, they are unable to live without water. If faced with a drought, and not able to bury themselves deep enough to remain in a wet place, they inevitably perish.

To properly care for leeches in household conditions, it is imperative to keep them in water. If leeches are deprived of water, they will excrete more slime and become less suitable for medical use.

In a dark place during the day or at night, leeches prefer to sleep by resting slightly over the water surface. This allows them to breathe easier and avoid having to constantly balance and adjust as they do when fully submerged. This, in turn, contributes to a longer and healthier life. When observing leeches in a contained environment, such as glass jar, one can notice that they often attach to the wall of the jar right above the water surface, with the lower half of their bodies remaining submerged.

In nature, leeches rarely swim. Instead, they frequently attach to stems and leaves of water plants where they await their prey. At night, they lie motionless, compressed into a ball while clinging to a plant or a stone. During cold, windy, or rainy weather, they sink to the bottom of the river or lake. Before a thunderstorm, they may become restless and float to the water surface. Strong thunderstorms have a bad effect on leeches, and can even lead to their death.

When observing them in a glass jar, you can see that natural or artificial light awakens them as they start to slowly move, detaching from the glass jar, and submerging into the water to swim. As a general rule, hungry leeches move toward the light, while the ones that are full move away from it.

In the constant hunt for food, leeches react to the prey's movement and heat. Leeches possess the sense of smell, taste, and touch. They also have numerous sensors, especially on the front part of the body, that help them locate their prey. Even insignificant movement in the water is enough to attract a hungry leech. *(Note: Usually, leeches do not react to the blood coming out of a wound of an animal, but they will quickly stick to the wound itself.)*

Almost any kind of sound can attract the attention of a hungry leech. But if sounds do not turn into a meal, these occurrences can further add to their hunger and loss of weight.

Historical Note: In 19th century Russia, watchmen were forbidden to use noisemakers for the purpose of scaring thieves and robbers around places where leeches were being raised because it would wake them up and disrupt their rest.

During the winter, leeches curl up and shrink into small balls while losing their sensitivity as they become less aware of their environment. Leeches can withstand cold winters fairly easily, and mature leeches can do it better than the young ones. They freeze as the water does and, as the water thaws out in the spring, they wake up, as energetic as ever. The leech has a special chemical in its tissues that protects it from water crystallization. But most of the time, during the winter, leeches bury themselves deep into the ground, curled up into a ball with the head inserted into the tail pit, and spend their entire winter dormant until it is warm again.

Leeches consume food in a liquid state, and nature has equipped them with a taste for more than just blood. While in cocoons, baby leeches eat the organic matter inside it. Once outside, they eat the slime on water plants, larvas of water insects, small snails, and worms. Mature leeches have a completely different diet though. Since they can bite through skin of a human or even thicker skin of other animals, they prefer to consume blood. Leeches have such a large appetite for blood that they have the ability to continue sucking even when their last meal has yet to be digested.

A medicinal leech can suck blood from any vertebrate species, including cattle, horses, and people. If they extract a crucial amount of blood, their victim may die; therefore, leeches are viewed as predators. For them, fish and frogs are just secondary supply of food; reptiles are almost insignificant and only fall prey to leeches under the extreme conditions.

It has been frequently observed that most adult leeches would reject any food other than blood. Perhaps, that is why they are able to wait for an extended period of time until a suitable meal comes along. This ability to fast for a long time has its price, though. In clean waters, a starving leech quickly becomes lean and may lose up to a quarter of its body weight in a year.

But even if it is content to extract other nutrients from surrounding water, it cannot fast forever. As its hunger grows, so does its aggression. A hungry leech will jump on every moving object, even if it is a passing stick (or even a corpse), although detaching almost immediately. Starving leeches will even attack well-fed leeches, hoping to extract blood from their stomach sacs, despite the fact that the blood inside of a leech changes over time and takes on a foul odor. These attacks often lead to wounds and even deaths. Cannibalism among leeches, however, is rare and is solely driven by extreme hunger.

Leeches are equipped with wide stomach pouches that act as food reserves for long periods of time. It takes a minimum of six months for a leech to digest its food. Out of all the leeches, the one that can endure hunger the longest without perishing is the medicinal leech—*Hirudo medicinalis*. This particular leech has received some attention from scientists just for having the ability to go without food from one to three years.

When food supplies within the digestive tract are exhausted, the tissues of the leech become more compact and filled with complex compounds that simulate the process of eating and allow them to go without food. Hungry leeches grow slowly. Therefore, in artificial conditions, it is imperative to feed them regularly so that they can reach the necessary size faster. And just from one feeding, a leech can gain five to seven times its own body weight.

A leech has to go through a lot to survive; so, nature has equipped it with a great food processing system. But it does not have a hard shell for protection or any poisonous excretions that may deter predators. This lacking in defense attracts many predators looking for an easy meal, including muskrats, water rats, otters, hedgehogs, minks, auks, turtles, certain fish, some worms, and water spiders.

Leeches today, however, face an even greater threat. Due to the considerable deterioration of the natural environment in the last few decades, some types of leeches are nearing a complete extinction. The situation is made worse by the artificial drainage of natural moors and reserves, chemical runoffs, and fishermen who use them for bait (even though they are on the endangered species list). At this time, it seems that only a higher awareness and the revival of leech therapy can contribute to an increase in the population of leeches. Otherwise, leeches are going to disappear from freshwater reservoirs just like they did in the middle of the last century in Western Europe, despite being actively protected by laws and regulations.

Meanwhile, raising leeches in an artificial environment presents its own challenges. Leech owners soon learn that, just like with people, it is much easier to prevent a disease than to cure it. By knowing what conditions enhance leeches' health—such as maintaining the correct temperature, proper lighting, feeding routines, handling and general care—you can considerably reduce their mortality rate.

The process of transplanting leeches from one environment to the other is not an easy one. Most leeches are caught in freshwater and then cultivated in laboratories following a specially-developed process, which takes approximately one year. First, a leech is caught in a natural setting and delivered to the lab. There, it is washed, quarantined, and fed with cow's blood. If babies are born, they are fed as well. When leeches are ready, they undergo a three to five month fasting process before being certified. And only then they become available for safe use.

Today, most laboratories focus on growing healthy leeches at a faster pace. With more encouraging results in the lab, and a greater awareness of medicinal leech's benefits, one day we may witness its return as a common medical treatment.

4

Leech Care

Selecting a quality leech

Leeches provide us with many health benefits and a unique medical means. They make an impact quickly and on many different levels. In the meantime, we have an obligation to preserve all fine and delicate facets of the leech's organism so that it can, in turn, deliver the appropriate care for us. Therefore, it is very important to know how to select healthy leeches and properly care for these wonderful little creatures.

Only use leeches from a trustworthy source that specializes in breeding and growing leeches certified for medical purposes. These leeches should come with certifications that reflect proper standards of health, size, age, and hunger level.

It is very risky to purchase leeches that were caught in the wild as well as attempting to catch leeches by yourself, since you do not want to contribute to the their extinction. Besides, leeches that are sourced from a natural setting might be contaminated by environmental pollutants (such as chemical runoffs, radiation, etc.) which may diminish their healing power or worsen the patient's condition.

The medicinal leech, *Hirudo medicinalis*, is usually the best choice. At the same time, the common leech, *Hirudo Officinalis*, may be better suited for certain illnesses for it bites deeper and causes more bleeding (although it takes a little bit longer to attach).

When purchasing leeches, always consider their age, size, and the state of health. Take your time to carefully observe their behaviors, whether in a jar or in nature. You do not want to choose those lying on the bottom, nor the ones curled up in a ball or a circle. Sometimes leeches remain still: some may be completely extended and motionless and some could be resting in a contorted position. To determine whether these leeches are unhealthy or just sleeping stir the water lightly and watch them in motion. Healthy and hungry leeches should start to swim almost immediately and move around with a great amount of energy.

Things to look for in a healthy leech:

- A great extension and becoming thin like worms when stretched out, while also able to fully contract to a great thickness.
- Rings that stack on top of each other smoothly and then quickly extend again.
- Plump backs and flat stomachs.
- During movement the tip of the head will become pointy and cone-like.
- Front and back suckers look like distinct mounds with layers that fluctuate in size like an accordion.

Characteristics of a healthy hungry leech prior to therapy:

- An increase in movement in response to disturbance.
- Positioning of the rings (smoothly overlapping, with no intervals).
- Elasticity of the body.
- Should be more flat, rather than a rounded form.
- Twisting the body in reaction to the human touch. The more the leech is able to curl up, the stronger it is. Under the fingers, it takes the form of an olive or a small cucumber, showing strength through the contraction of its body, and further

displaying elasticity. On the other hand, the less elastic, soft, lazy, slow moving leeches are the ones that can be categorized as either full (from a meal) or unhealthy. These categories of leeches never stretch to full length and the intervals between the rings are very noticeable.

- If let out into a vessel with small amount of water, the healthy leech will make its way to the top in less than half an hour and stay there.
- If taken out of the water and placed on a hard dry surface, it moves quickly using its front and back suckers.
- If you submerge your hand in the water, the healthy leech immediately tries to attach to it.

Containers

The key to success begins with having a well-maintained storage. There are different materials to choose from, but glass and clay containers work the best. In the past, wooden containers were used as well.

You can choose from small to large jars, pots, jugs, etc. But keep in mind that the optimal water volume for one leech is from 40 to 120 ml; therefore a small space, such as a three-liter jug filled halfway with water, should not house more than fifty leeches. And you should never keep more than ten leeches in a one-liter jar.

Just as the container size varies from one to the next, so does the care for leeches. And different specialists will employ different techniques. But regardless of what technique is used, remember that while caring for medicinal leeches is not difficult, it does require following basic guidelines for diligent care and cleanliness.

Young and vigorous leeches of average size may share the same place, but the slower moving leeches and the ones that curl into a ball should be held separately until they recover. A good rule of thumb is to observe the overall health of leeches in one jar. If you notice that one is sick, you should immediately separate it from the rest to make sure that the others do not become ill as well.

In nature, leeches thrive in fast-moving freshwater streams. When using leeches for medical purposes, it is essential to ensure that the conditions of the artificial environment mirror their natural habitat as much as possible, whether they are kept in a small jar or a large tank for breeding. You can use tap water, but only after it has been left to settle for a few days. The best water for leeches, however, is from a lake, river, or collected rain water. In any case, you should never use boiled water. And do not use well water since it may contain particles that can irritate your leeches causing them to attack each other, with sometimes fatal results.

When preparing a container, fill it with water halfway, or up to two-thirds. When you place leeches in one container, you may notice that, within the first few days, the water turns green due to their excretions. This is a good sign of their healthy conditions.

Clean environment

It is essential for a leech to live in a clean and comfortable environment. To keep leeches healthy, change water regularly, with new water not being lower in temperature than the old one. During winter, change water weekly; in the summer, two times a week; and during great heat, daily. Also, water should be changed if you notice that it has turned dark-green due to excessive slime, has some brownish stains, and/or a thin layer of skin shed by the leech is floating on the surface.

Changing water should be done very carefully because it is always very stressful for the leech. You can empty the contents one of two ways: 1) use a sponge to absorb the old water, or 2) pour out the entire contents into a strainer while leaving the attached leeches in the jar. Then, gently rinse the leeches to get rid of excess slime. This step is important because the accumulated slime can block leeches' respiratory passages and may cause them to get ill, or even die. If you need to transfer leeches from one container to the next, use a wooden spoon to limit human contact.

If you are to store leeches in a container for an extended period of time with limited maintenance, place clean sand and small pieces of charcoal on the bottom of the container so that a leech can use them to clean itself. The same can be achieved by water plants, such as *Equisetum palustre* (marsh horsetail), *Myriophyllum verticillatum* (whorled water milfoil), *Potamogeton natans* (broad-leaved pondweed), and others. This way, you can store a small number of leeches (around ten) for up to a year with little or no upkeep.

Unhealthy leech

A dead or unhealthy leech should be immediately removed from the jar, so that the others are not infected or harmed by the spoiled water. A sick leech can be easily spotted because it lies stretched out on the bottom of the container and excretes brownish slime with white grains. You may also notice that it will hardly respond to your touch when picked up to be removed from the container.

Additional care tips

Leeches usually handle gradual fluctuations in temperature better than drastic changes. Young leeches can adapt easier to higher temperatures, while the older ones are better at adapting to colder temperatures. Although in extreme situations they are able to survive in temperatures as high as 100° F and as low as 20° F, the optimal range is between 40 and 55° F. And do not allow the temperature to fall below 37° F, or leeches may freeze.

For the optimal living conditions store leeches in cool places in the summer and frequently take the container outside to provide them with fresh air. During the winter, it is best to keep them in a warm room. The air in the room or storage area should be clean, especially during winter, and free of any noticeable odors, including tobacco smoke. Keep the container in a quiet place because too much noise can disturb leeches and, if they are hungry, lead to their exhaustion and weight loss.

To protect leeches from constant light exposure, place a removable cover on the container or paint the bottom half with black paint.

Always cover the jar with natural fabrics, such as linen, and secure it with a rubber band. Do not forget to check that air can get in and out; otherwise, leeches will suffocate. Make sure that you are using a sufficiently strong fabric because leeches can chew through thinner gauze-like materials and crawl out.

Errors to avoid

- Full (fed) leeches, or ones that just drunk blood but have been manually drained, should never be in the same container with hungry leeches.

- Avoid using chemical cleaners to clean the container. Instead, rinse it thoroughly with running water.

- One of the more common errors in leech care is adding to the water unnecessary substances, such as sugar, honey, or even blood in an attempt to boost leeches' health or try to prevent their death. This practice should be avoided because it will actually have the opposite effect on leeches and not only contaminate the water but can also contribute to their illnesses and even death, especially in the summer.

5

Leech Therapy Process

Learning and understanding

When it comes to leech therapy, the importance of being thorough and detail-oriented should never be underestimated. A comfortable environment should be created not only for the patient, but also for the hard working leech.

Although practitioners can see the incredible advantages of leech therapy for patients, their families and the leech population, it is often difficult to introduce this approach into modern medicine. So, starting from the very first treatment, the specialist should carefully consider the condition of the patient and inform the patient (and his family) about various treatment tactics and therapy options. Techniques as to how to attach a leech and the process of detaching a leech and removing blood from it following the treatment should also be discussed. Afterwards, the patient should be allowed to take a leech home in a jar, along with the proper instructions of care, so he can increase his comfort level by becoming more familiar with the creature.

Psychological preparation

The specialist should carefully explain the process, emphasizing leech's inability to cause harm, and make sure that the patient completely understands the procedure, the health benefits of the treatment, and is psychologically ready to embrace leech therapy.

Positive attitude and understanding goes a long way. Very often patients are not only indifferent to, or ignorant of, the benefits of leeches, but they may also have negative emotions (and even hate) towards leeches. They may experience discomfort, even fear, around these little healers. In such cases, one should not expect to achieve any great outcomes from therapy sessions. If the patient does not understand or accept the method of healing presented to him by the doctor, he may not achieve the desired results. Therefore, in addition to its physiological effects, the possible psychological effects of leech therapy on the patient should be carefully examined.

When the specialist has decided to use leech therapy, the first step is to reinforce the morale of the patient—especially women, children, elderly, and anyone new to the process. It is necessary to calm and encourage them; and thoroughly explain the process while drawing on previous successful examples of using a leech as a natural approach to healing. The patient should embrace leech therapy and look forward to the treatment with excitement and enthusiasm, especially if sessions are to be repeated several times.

Getting started

Sessions should be conducted in a clean, preferably sterile, environment. The person administering the therapy should have clean dry hands. All clothing should be as odor-free as possible and not have any strong smells such as tobacco, cologne, or alcohol. The air should be fresh and warm, especially during the cold time of year.

The patient should be advised to bathe before a session (if possible), or to take extra efforts to clean themselves prior to therapy (especially the genital region if treatment will be in that area). The use of harsh or strongly-scented cleaners should be avoided.

In most instances, the patient should not eat before a leech therapy session. It is a good idea to clean out the intestines with the help of fiber or an enema prior to the procedure and use the bathroom right before to the session begins.

Because a large portion of the patient's body may be exposed (or bare) during the procedure, the specialist should ensure that the room is free of drafts and has a nice comfortable temperature.

The patient should be positioned on a clean cover topped off with a sterile sheet or a towel to absorb any water and blood that may seep during the procedure.

If leeches will be applied on a hairy spot of the body, shave the area and clean it with water and odorless soap. Use a wipe soaked in burdock oil to remove all traces of ointments, band aids, or developing pus, and then again wash and pat it dry with a cotton ball.

If the skin is cold or rigid, a hot compress consisting of a well wrung out towel, that was submerged in water of 120° F may be applied until the patient feels that it has cooled. Then, the skin is once again wiped down with hot water and dried. This warming of the skin is done not only to draw blood to the surface, but also to open up and clean skin pores. To achieve the same result, you may rub the skin with a soft cloth until the skin turns red and the patient experiences a warm sensation.

Try to schedule sessions in the evening, close to the bedtime, so that the patient may get a good night's sleep following the treatment. But if it is not possible—any time is fine, as long as the patient is fully informed about the treatment and its possible aftereffects.

Before starting a session, make sure that several items are readily available and accessible, such as: clean hot water in a small tub; a new, unused sponge; sterile gauze, cotton balls, band aids and bandages; sterilized tweezers; hygienic trays, test tubes or small jars.

During the procedure the patient can rest in any position, as long as he is comfortable enough to remain still throughout the process, which may take anywhere from a half to one and a half hours. The patient can be in a seated position during time of attachment and then lay down for the remaining part of the session, especially if feeling weak and short-winded. *(Note: If the leech is placed around the anus, then the patient should never be in a seated position.)*

After proper preparations, you may begin the session using one or several leeches simultaneously. Working with leeches requires experience, which can be acquired during the first few sessions while under the care of a professional. Until then, you should only undergo treatments with an experienced specialist.

General guidelines:

- Hungry and healthy leeches may be used at any time of day without any harm to the person, or the leech itself.
- When preparing for a session, remember that the leech intended to be used that day should be separated from the other leeches and placed in cold water.
- It is good to have twice the amount of leeches prepared than you actually intend to use. This precaution is necessary because individual leeches attach differently to the various parts of the body and may have unique reactions to each patient.
- To save time during the procedure, it is recommended to take the leech out of the container right before the treatment and place them in an empty glass jar or a test tube, which later can also be used to attach the leech to the patient.
- Some also recommend that, after taking it out of its container and prior to using it, one should gently wipe the leech with a cloth, while others disagree and believe that it irritates the leech, and, in some instances, may lead to negative outcomes (such as a leech's inability to attach).

Where to apply

In leech therapy, most specialists and doctors follow the rule of thumb: *place the leech where it hurts.* However, in practice, it is not all that simple. Deciding on the exact placement can be quite tricky.

Factors to consider:

- Patients themselves (age, health, etc.);
- The nature of the ailment;
- How long the patient has been suffering prior to treatment.

To achieve the desired results, take a special care to review all these factors. *(Note: Chapter 7 maps out the exact placement and quantity of leeches for specific illnesses, based on the information that has been documented by many doctors who have been healing patients with leech therapy.)*

There is a growing number of observers and doctors who feel that, contrary to common beliefs, the leech does not have to be positioned over the suffering organ only, but may be applied far away from the affected area and still be effective. However, this opinion has not been completely validated by a sufficient number of facts or studies.

Based on clinical evidence, some doctors also believe that the main benefit of leeches is not the amount of blood that they extract, but their ability to suck it from deeper parts of the person's body. But again, these ideas are just developing and still require more clinical evidences.

In the 1940's, S.Zaslavsky documented how to achieve an extraction of blood not just from the surface, but from the deeper parts of the body. This research made connections between the microcirculation system, blood vessels, lymph vessels, the nerve system under the skin and within the bodies of humans and animals. His studies opened doors for developing a system of placement during therapy that would achieve a blood flow not only on the surface but from the depths of the organism.

Unfortunately, a big portion of this work went unrecognized by the mainstream medical community. Nevertheless, some private practitioners were able to use this information and claim to achieve great results in dealing with many specific illnesses and general poor health.

During the last few years, leech therapy has expanded to include the mapping of certain points of placement on the body that correlate to specific diseases, although experience with this type of approach is still fairly limited. With more work being done and documented, people will soon be able to fully appreciate the great benefits of this approach.

Note about placement order: In certain cases, the order of points of attachment becomes important. For example, if leeches are attached vertically, then it is better to start from the bottom and work your way up. This way, the already-attached leeches are not interfering with the newly-placed ones.

How many to use

Another tricky aspect of leech therapy is determining the number of leeches to use during the treatment. The most commonly used standard is 2-5-7-10, or even 15-20, leeches per treatment. But if you stop to think about it for a moment, it is not entirely clear why this number should produce the best results.

Not long ago, traditional leech specialists routinely recommended one leech per two pounds of body weight. This calculation results in the application of fifteen to twenty leeches per session. And over the course of four or five sessions, even with breaks of seven to eight days in between, it could easily amount to a hundred leeches total. Unfortunately, these high-quantity leech treatments may have a negative impact on an older person or a patient with a weaker immune system, or when optimal results can be achieved with much fewer leeches.

In each particular case, it is better to work off the individual instead off a set number. Before deciding on the quantity of leeches and sessions, the specialist should carefully consider the patient's age, sex, physical condition, overall strength, irritability towards leeches, the progression of their disease, surrounding climate, time of year, the quality of the air, room temperature, etc. Likewise, the volume of the extracted blood will depend on the leeches' types, size, health, and level of hunger. All these factors should be considered in addition to the amount of bleeding after the removal of a leech, and whether you should take off the leeches early or let them fall off on their own.

Given that so many different factors should be taken into consideration, it is often difficult to set one universal standard for the quantity of leeches to be used in each particular case. Therefore, choosing the right number of leeches for a specific therapy session will depend on the experience and intuition of the specialist who should be able to consider all the relevant (and irrelevant) factors.

In any case, the specialist should not attempt to establish a cookie-cutter blueprint for all cases by "standardizing" the quantity of leeches per session. It must be recognized that approaches and methods of this therapy will vary with each individual patient and each specific illness.

How long does it last?

There are two primary approaches:

- Let leeches feed until they are full and fall off by themselves. This usually takes about 30 minutes to 2 hours.
- Leeches are allowed to penetrate the skin and then taken off by the specialist almost immediately, followed by open bleeding from the wound. This method usually involves a much higher quantity of leeches, and blood-letting happens without the leeches consuming any blood.

The mechanics of attachment

The modern style of attaching a leech does not present any serious challenges because most leeches are quite willing to stick to any part of the body, with the exception of the palms of the hands and soles of the feet (although even this can be accomplished if absolutely necessary). Remember, however, that leeches are sensitive to different parts of the body, skin thickness, the patient's sex and age, how close the blood vessels are to the surface, etc.

In general, leeches attach faster and easier to soft skin rather than to the coarse and thick type. Leeches seem to favor women over men and prefer children to adults. When a leech attaches in less-favorable conditions, it will bite less and more shallow resulting in less outflow of blood.

To derive maximum benefits of leech therapy, it is imperative to understand how the leech attaches itself and extracts blood. This knowledge should also help you to recognize why claims that leeches cause infections are completely unfounded. In addition, you must gain a general understanding of how to treat individual cases, physical and biological properties of leeches, treatment details, and many different ways of using leech therapy, either by itself or in conjunction with other methods.

The medicinal leech has three jaws—all of which are equipped with pointy, sharp, little teeth. It is this efficient mechanism that allows the leech to bite through the skin, other soft tissues, or mucous membranes.

After it attaches to the chosen point of a body, the leech then extends its suction cup and narrows its lips, protruding them beyond its jaws, creating a vacuum effect as it suctions onto the skin. During this process, the skin of the patient (or prey) is pulled towards its teeth as the muscles around its lips continue to tighten. The leech uses its strongest and sharpest front teeth to make the first cut through the skin. Next, the leech uses all three jaws, which resemble semicircular saws, to further penetrate the skin. A patient usually feels a pull or suction, at the spot of the cupping, followed by a little bit of discomfort or pain while the skin is being pierced.

After forming an open wound, in the shape of an upside down Y inside of a circle, the leech proceeds to suck blood. During this process, the saliva secreted through its salivary glands passes through an opening between the front teeth and into the wound. This saliva contains many biologically-active substances, including a numbing agent, which reduces the pain of the bite, and hirudin, which prevents the blood from clotting.

During the entire process, the leech moves and wiggles, using the rings on its body for balance and support. As it contracts and expands, it is an indication that a healthy stream of blood is being extracted by the leech. Over time, the rings gradually expand, starting from the back end and becoming smoother and more even. Meanwhile, the body of a leech becomes heavy, and starts to excrete quite a bit of slime. After becoming full, the leech lets go and falls off on its own.

Once the leech has detached, bleeding from the bite may continue up to twenty-four hours, primarily because the walls of the wound and the nearby blood vessels have been coated with hirudin from the leech's saliva. Treating this bleeding is easy, but requires a few key steps which are described later.

> *Note about infection: Once you understand how the leech functions, it should become clear that it is impossible for it to transfer any infection or poison, even if it were concentrated in its mouth. This is mostly due to the process of contraction and expansion of the body which creates a vacuum effect and prevents any original blood from reentering the wound. As a result, the leech is virtually incapable of infecting its supplier.*

Can't get it to stick

It is best if the leech attaches quickly and naturally. However, there are cases when leeches, despite all your efforts and care, do not want to attach. Before ruling these leeches out as unfit for the treatment, there are a few ways you can lure them to do the job.

A few tricks of the trade include:

- Grasp the front end of the leech with two fingers and hold it next to the skin until it attaches. If necessary, this can be repeated with all the leeches during a session. You may also hold a leech using a pair of tweezers, but keep in mind that it may irritate the leech. A distressed or irritated leech will start to wiggle or move around on the skin of the patient, and most likely will never attach.
- Although not very convenient, another method is to put a leech in a test tube with the tail end of the leech towards the bottom and the head facing the opening of the tube. Then flip the tube upside down on top of the intended area and hold it in place until the leech attaches. *(Note: This is the only way to place a leech on mucous membranes.)*
- One or several leeches may also be placed in a small glass or jar. The jar is turned over onto the skin in the intended treatment area and held in place until leeches attach. If a leech starts crawling up the side of the jar, just give it a shake until it falls down. Keep the jar in place until all leeches (if more than one) have attached themselves. (This is a great method to use with children and adults who are afraid of leeches.)
- A close alternative to this method is to put a small piece of linen in a glass or a jar so that the corners are sticking out. Place the leeches into the container. Then press the glass against the body tight enough so that the leeches cannot escape. Gradually pull at the corners of the linen. As the area gets smaller and smaller, the leeches become pressed to the body and are left with no option but to quickly attach.
- Take a sheet of paper and cut out holes where you wish the leeches to attach, thus, creating a blueprint where you want to concentrate your

therapy. Turn over the glass with the leeches onto the sheet of paper. Since leeches feel uncomfortable on the paper they will quickly find the holes and make their attachments. Once the leeches have attached, you can remove the glass but keep the paper in place since you have to keep either gauze or a sheet between the leeches and the patient's skin anyway so that their lower body movements do not annoy the patient and to prevent them from attaching their bottom suckers to the skin.

If all methods described previously had failed, you may use a variety of baits to lure the leech. Sweets, milk, water diluted with sugar, egg yolk, or other things that are pleasant and refreshing to leeches may be rubbed onto the skin. Pricking the skin with a needle and allowing a few drops of blood to come out, while rubbing it into the skin, may also attract a reluctant leech.

If these methods still do not work, you can use materials that irritate the leech, such as wine or apple juice, because, while trying to escape, the leech will instinctively bite and attach to the skin.

Another way is to place the leech in some irritant for about five minutes prior to the session and then, after taking it out, gently rinse it with warm water (not higher than 65° F) and place it on the skin using the simple methods described previously.

The use of irritants was first introduced by the English and the procedure was performed with a glass filled one-quarter of the way with water and the necessary quantity of leeches. Then the glass was pressed tightly onto the patient's skin in the intended area. If leeches attempted to crawl up the glass, it was repeatedly shaken so that they ended up falling to the skin and became submerged in water.

Although this method was labor intensive, it was very effective, and the leeches bit through the skin almost immediately, with minimal pain felt by the patient. As soon as all of the leeches were attached, a towel was positioned to absorb the water around the glass which was slowly lifted up. Then both were removed to leave the leeches to complete their work.

Today, a variation of this English method includes a one-to-one mixture of water and wine. The strong smell of wine irritates the leech and causes it to try to escape by biting through the skin even faster.

Leeches can also be attached using an apple by carving a hole in it, placing the leech inside, and pressing it on the skin. The acidity of the apple juice motivates the leech to try to escape and, as a result, it attaches to the skin quickly.

On occasion, the selected leeches do not react to alcohol, sour sources, or even sweets. Usually this is a sign of poor quality of leeches, and that they should be replaced immediately.

What to do after the leech has attached

After having found a convenient place on the skin, the leech will stop and bite through it. As soon as the leech has attached, the container used for attachment is immediately removed. When fully attached, the leech pauses for a moment, its head widens as it becomes compressed with the neck, and then it begins to feed. During this process the leech's body expands and contracts in a wavy motion when it swallows the blood and moves it from the front to the tail end of the body. These movements continue until the leech is full. If you had little prior experience with leeches, it is difficult sometimes to distinguish the front end and back end of the leech. But if you look closely for this wavy movement, you will be able to tell them apart quite easily.

It is important to note that, normally, the leech not only uses the front sucker to attach, but also the back one. Since it can weaken the leech's ability to extract blood, you may want to carefully disconnect the back sucker from the skin. But do not use your hands to partially detach a leech because you may tear off a part of the front sucker and expose the wound to possible infections. Instead, use a method that is similar to early termination of attachment that includes applying salt, tobacco leaves or other irritants, such as vinegar and lemon juice (discussed in detail in the next few pages). After detaching the rear sucker, place a cotton ball, gauze, or a clean sheet of paper between the leech's lower body and the patient's skin. That way the patient will not be annoyed by the leech's movements or disgusted by the slime it excretes when feeding.

During the session, it is important not to disturb the leech because it can detach prematurely, without having accomplished its full medical purpose. Also, an overly irritated leech may throw up the blood it just consumed. If a leech attaches itself but falls off prior to swallowing blood, you may replace it with another one by positioning it right on the same spot.

In some cases, a leech begins the session well by actively sucking blood, but then abruptly slows down, and even stops, almost like freezing in place or falling asleep. To "revive" the leech, gently wipe it from front to back with a cotton ball soaked in warm water. If the leech does not react to this treatment, then you may consider it defective and replace it with a fresh one. As a rule of thumb, though, it is better to leave leeches alone until they become full and fall off on their own.

During the feeding process, the body of the leech will increase in length, volume, and weight. As the leech gradually becomes full, the increased weight of its own body will pull it down off the patient's skin. To prevent it from falling off too early and/or causing pain to the patient, place a piece of fabric underneath the leech for support. Under the right circumstances, as its body expands and the leech falls, it will leave a wound that continues to bleed.

How to detach leeches

Occasionally, a leech remains attached for a long time, even after it has stopped consuming blood. In these instances, there are several methods to terminate a treatment:

- Cover the leech with salt, tobacco leaves, or ash (from wood);
- Spray it with saltwater;
- Blow tobacco smoke at it;
- Apply an irritant such as vinegar, wine, lemon juice, and urine.

If all these methods don't work, use a scalpel to carefully detach the leech's upper lip from the skin. When the air enters between the skin and the sucker, it should break the vacuum/suction and cause the leech's front sucker to detach. Be careful not to cut nor sever the body of the leech itself because it will not yield any results and the leech may even continue to suck blood.

Although there are many ways of detaching a leech artificially, these methods are still inferior to the natural way of a leech falling off on its own.

How much blood?

How much blood extraction is healthy? This question has been asked since ancient times and, even today, doctors and researchers still disagree on this subject. So, is it really possible to know exactly how much blood is extracted during a session? Yes, but only if all leeches were all of the same type and size, were all equally hungry or equally full after consuming an equal amount of blood. But even then, with most things being identical, some leeches tend to stay attached for over an hour, while others fall off after only a few minutes having consumed almost nothing at all. And how would you estimate the subsequent bleeding which may continue for half an hour or longer (with rare cases being even close to twenty-four hours)?

If you had the opportunity to observe twenty similar treatments, you would find that perhaps only two had similar volumes of blood extracted, while even bleeding from the same wound varies from one session to the next. This inconsistency in the volume of blood that leaves the body is one of the major drawbacks of leech therapy because it requires close attention of a specialist, who can monitor the amount of blood extracted and make decisions with regard to the continuation of treatment, cessation of the procedure, improvement in health, or any discomfort the patient may be experiencing.

There are many factors that affect the amount of blood that leaves the body during a session. For once, it has been observed that the speed of suction depends on several conditions: time of year the leech was acquired; transportation and storage method afterwards; its age, size, health, and energy; etc. It has also been documented that larger leeches consume slower and fall off quicker, while the smaller ones are weaker and extract even less blood. In contrast, the medium-size leeches of average strength eagerly consume until they are completely full (and even in rare occasions, until they are fatally full).

This inability to determine the amount of blood extracted by a leech is further complicated by several other issues. For example, leeches are greatly affected by seasonal changes and temperature fluctuations. Strong summer heat and severe winter frosts often have a crippling effect on leeches. On the positive note, they are often in great shape during the fall, and feel even better in the spring.

The degree of a leech's hunger will also determine its appetite for blood. A full leech is less enthusiastic than a hungry one. Hungry leeches act very aggressively to satisfy their needs, although overly-exhausted leeches are incapable of operating normally. Keep in mind that leeches are able to lose up to seventy-five percent of their mass when starved for extended period of time, which may leave them without energy and unable to extract blood.

Yet another factor that affects the volume of blood is the leech's reaction to the patient. As any other living being, leeches react differently to a patient's age, condition of the vascular system, condition of the skin, etc. The thin and fresh skin of children (of either sex) is highly appealing to a leech, whereas the weak, old, poorly-circulated skin of the elderly decreases its aggressiveness and eagerness to stick to the body. Specific placement on the body also matters. Leeches prefer biting through skin on the neck as well as any other places where there is more blood circulation in the capillaries.

The medical leech weighs about 3 grams and can extract about 15 ml of blood within a half an hour to an hour before detachment. Afterwards, the wound may release almost an equal amount of blood. The existing empirical evidences indicate that during a procedure anywhere from 12 to 30 ml of blood is released from the body. *(Note: Other studies have shown that the volume can reach as high as 60 ml).*

High-quality, artificially-grown leeches demonstrate very consistent performances and act in a more similar manner than the ones captured in the wild. This performance consistency of the lab-grown leeches helps to eliminate a small portion of the volume-guessing game. Moreover, unlike the ones captured in nature, lab-grown leeches are completely safe to use.

> *General guidelines: If a patient requires a minimal blood*
> *extraction, then it is better to use younger, smaller leeches.*
> *If a greater volume is needed, medium and large leeches*
> *are better.*

What happens to the blood?

Does the blood extracted by a leech differ from the blood extracted by other means? As early as the 1800's doctors suspected that, because the leech extracts blood from small blood vessels and capillaries, this blood must be different than the blood let out through the larger veins.

Moreover, in the past, it was thought that the consumed blood does not change, since it remained undigested and in the same liquid state even after a long period of time. But when researches used the same leeches and squeezed the blood out of them after feeding, it became evident that the blood coming directly from the veins is different from that in leeches' stomachs. The vein's blood quickly clotted, while the blood extracted from leeches remained liquid and homogeneous.

In 1902, the substance hirudin was discovered (hirudo means leech in Latin). As research progressed, even more enzymes and biological components were discovered within the blood. More importantly, the symbiotic bacteria *Bacillus Hirudiensie* had been found inside the leech itself. It has been shown to kills microbes in the leech's intestines and in the digested blood. This discovery provided further support to the notion that leeches grown in lab environments are unable to infect a person during leech therapy.

To bleed or not to bleed

Each patient will seek different results from leech therapy. With that in mind, here are a few approaches to choose from:

- Leave the wound to bleed freely for the amount of time determined by the specialist.
- Artificially help the wound bleed more. This method is better suited for traditional methods: hot compresses made from various materials such as flax seeds, hot soaked white bread, or hot milk. Hot water may be applied as well. When compresses cool, exchange them for the hot ones. You may also rinse the wounds using water with a temperature of up to 100° F and position the wound over the steam coming off the hot water. Submerging the treated body part in a hot bath will also encourage bleeding. Cupping (*a method of placing cups with reduced air pressure on the skin to create suction*) can be used as well. Whatever method you choose, bleeding should continue until the blood color changes from dark red to light red.
- Stop the bleeding as soon as possible. This happens more often when treating the elderly, children, and women who have weaker skin. Or when an inexperienced specialist may have placed a leech over a vein or an artery (which are easily punctured by the leech's teeth, resulting in excessive bleeding). Therefore, it is important for the specialist to stay with the patient until the bleeding has ceased completely.

After the session

Each patient should strictly follow their individual instructions for what to do after a therapy session. This plan is usually created after the procedure when the specialist has had the ability to observe the organism's reaction to the treatment and has fully gauged the patient's condition.

In most cases, for faster healing, the patient should remain at home. If two or three leeches were applied, the patient should rest for one day. When a higher quantity of leeches is used, the patient may need to rest one to two days (or longer) depending on the disease and resulting condition of the patient.

Patients will be able to take full baths in five to six days; although, within a day, they are typically able to take a cool to warm shower.

> *Note: It is recommended to avoid using other medicines not only following the procedure, but (especially) during leech therapy because the medicine can interfere with your ability to judge the effectiveness of the treatment.*

Even prior to the leech falling off, there may be redness and swelling where the mouth of the leech is attached to the skin. It will become even more prominent after the leech falls off. The teeth make a mark that looks like an upside down "Y". Its size ranges from 1 to 2 mm in diameter, with a depth of 1.5 mm. The wound itself looks like a precise incision that continues to bleed from the Y-shape.

The skin around the wound may also become bruised and turn dark blue as a consequence of the suction process. It will then turn yellow and remain so for about two weeks. Gradually, the skin returns to its normal color. Depending on the patient, the wound may also heal as a Y-shaped scar, become white in color, and remain visible for a few years.

Some patients may feel hot or experience a rise in temperature. The pain and discomfort, in this instance, is usually experienced for about twelve hours. Sometimes, it can even last up to twenty-four hours. But, in most cases, it subsides hour by hour.

It is quite normal to experience bleeding after the leech falls off, but it may range from a minimal amount to an amount that requires immediate intervention to stop it, especially if the patient is a child. Most wounds usually bleed for two to six hours, although bleeding may continue up to twenty-four hours, and sometimes even longer. But the entire duration of allowed bleeding should be decided by the specialist.

To stop the bleeding, the wound should be covered with a sterile bandage and, if necessary, tightly wrapped to apply extra pressure. Once the bandage is in place, the specialist should check it on a regular basis to make sure that the bleeding stopped. If, after leaving the office, the patient notices that blood is seeping through the bandage, another layer of dressing should be added over the old one, while still applying pressure on the wound.

Bandages should be changed daily, and the wound may be wiped with hydrogen peroxide. Other ways of stopping bleeding include the use of a grape vinegar compress, cold water compress, or even ice. If these methods do not provide the desired results, you may try using nitrate silver. To apply this method, use two fingers to spread the nitrate silver around the edges of the wound, wipe down the area with a cotton ball, and proceed to bandage the wound.

To stop bleeding from the gums, thoroughly rinse using a mixture of cold water and vinegar, or water that has been boiled with oak bark.

Possible complications

Although complications with leech therapy are very rare, it is necessary to be aware of them, along with ways to prevent and treat them. The specialist should make a point of constantly monitoring the patient and inquiring as to how they feel during the treatment. Remember, all individuals react in individual ways, but a good specialist should be able to build upon past medical experiences and results.

Seek the attention of a doctor immediately if you notice the following:

- The patient is turning pale.
- The patient is feeling faint, dizzy, or nauseous.
- The extremities become cold.
- The pulse begins to be rapid and/or weak.

(Note: A weak pulse is not always an indication that one should not conduct leech therapy and may actually mean quite the opposite, so this condition should be assessed on a case by case basis.)

Seek the attention of a doctor while still applying the basic methods to stop the bleeding. Under extreme circumstances, the doctor may be forced to stitch up the wound, although, when the wound is located at the extremities *(arms and legs)*, the doctor may choose to use a tourniquet.

Sometimes, the wound refuses to heal and it may be accompanied by pain, inflammation, and pus. This often depends on the nervous system, the sickness of the person, the nature of the disease, etc. However, more often than not, these cases are the results of improper care of the wound, or the specialist's use of irritants (such as the ones described earlier that include salts, acids, alcohol). It may also happen when the attached leech was continuously touched or disturbed while already attached, resulting in the leech vomiting blood back into the wound.

Another complication that the patient may experience is itching. Most often the itch is at the location of the wound, but, occasionally, the patient's the entire body may be itching. This itch may persist a day or two before going away on its own. (Of course, to avoid the risk of infection, the patient should never scratch the wounds).

If the patient has an especially itchy wound, she may rub it with a half-and-half mixture of ammonia and Vaseline. If this does not help, reapplying the leech to the same area may do the job. Also, to stop the itching, you may take a hot bath or use cupping *(placing jars with reduced air pressure on the skin to create suction)*.

To prevent the development of inflammation, gently rub the wound with white vinegar and apply cold water compresses. Bandages soaked with burdock oil or glycerine can help as well. If puffiness and redness develops, simply soak a towel in warm water (about 70° F) and apply it to the affected area. Wait until the towel loses its heat, and then repeat. *(Note: Usually, compresses are not done until it becomes imperative to see drastic results.)*

For especially strong inflammatory reactions, it is also possible to apply a cold compress. To do so, mix sea salt with water (one tablespoon per quart); take three towels and submerge them in the mixture; slightly wring out the towels; place the towels in individual plastic bags; and put them in a freezer for two to two and a half hours. Afterwards, take one towel out of the freezer, remove it from the plastic bag, and apply it directly to the affected area. As soon as it feels extremely cold, remove the towel. When the area regains its normal temperature, apply the next towel. Repeat the process with the third towel as well. To get the desired effect and reduce the inflammation, this process can be repeated as many times as necessary.

When allergic reactions and/or inflammations are mild, they usually do not need any major treatment; however, in rare cases it is possible to experience some skin inflammation with a higher degree of intensity in places where the skin may bubble up with blood, burst and break, leaving the wound wet and exposed.

A word of caution

It is very important for the specialist to have the right experience and intuition to understand the patient's needs before performing any services. Yet, as with any trade, there always those who are active in the practice even though they are causing more harm than good. Unfortunately, these careless few may inflict enough damage to discredit the entire profession of leech therapy and endanger the future of professionals who stand behind it.

It also doesn't help that leech therapy is frequently shunned by doctors who have modern training in medicine but have very little understanding of leeches, much less their healing benefits. These well-respected professionals spread the word that leeches cause diseases, or are ineffective. And because of their high social status, this verdict—although ignorant—carries a great deal of weight and is widely accepted in our culture without any questions.

In some instances, it is true that careless use of leeches can cause a great deal of harm. This may happen when a therapist looks to cure every disease with leeches, without examining the patient's condition more closely and realizing that it is impossible to treat everything at once. In these unfortunate cases, instead of curing the disease, the therapist often weakens the patient and decreases the chances of healing, which almost guarantees the treatment's failure.

Although most opposition to leech therapy has stemmed from only a few sources, some still insist that leech therapy may be harmful, especially when a patient's blood is already thin and unable to clot easily. They also point to other problems such as hemolysis (*the breakdown of red blood cells*), anaemia, shock to the organism, and possible allergic reactions to the treatment, while completely ignoring the fact that, in the hands of an expert, serious side effects of leech therapy are practically nonexistent.

Most leech therapists agree that if the treatment is done right and the patient diligently follows all instructions, then it should not be performed more than twice (or even once) a year. But beware of those who apply a great deal of leeches and conduct a large quantity of procedures that may weaken the body, lead to anemia, and, at times, result in hospitalization.

Mistakes to avoid

- Leech therapy is not suitable for patients diagnosed with hemophilia or anemia.
- Pregnant women should not use leech therapy.
- Since immune system stimulation is a big part of the leech therapy healing process, people with weak or deteriorated immune systems should check with their physicians.
- In rare cases, a leech can be mistakenly placed on a vein, resulting in a strong prolonged flow of purple-colored blood. If it is placed on an artery, there will be rhythmic gushing of bright red blood after the detachment of a leech. In either

case, the person is in serious danger and requires the immediate assistance of a doctor to close the wound and stop the blood loss.

- It is very important to be extremely cautious when using leech therapy to treat children and the elderly.
- A specialist should proceed with caution (not to mention the full disclosure and patient's consent) before placing leeches on mucous membranes such as the tongue and gums or the clitoral hood since the leech may penetrate deeper in those areas.
- In certain cases, it is strongly recommended to place leeches on the tailbone rather the anal opening. For once, it is easier to stop the bleeding around the tailbone. Also, it is less traumatic for the patient and will not interfere with the person's bowel movements in the future. And finally, the tailbone area is easier to clean before and after the procedure.
- One should be extremely careful when attaching leeches to the parts of the skin that shift with everyday bodily movements.
- Very thin skin, such as eyelids, cheeks, scrotum, etc., can easily swell up and bruise.
- Places where the blood vessels are right underneath the surface of the skin may bleed excessively.
- The punctured skin of the patient can show bruising for some time after a treatment. A few people may also be more prone to scarring and might develop small white scars in places where the skin was penetrated. In these cases, avoid using leeches on open areas of the body, including the neck, face, forearms, and the top part of the chest.

- It is a common mistake to use a large number
  of leeches (sometimes more than ten) without
  the supervision of a specialist. This can result
  in a great deal of harm from excessive blood loss
  and an unbalanced homeostasis of an organism,
  making a person even more vulnerable to the
  progression of a disease (or to acquiring a
  new one).

6

Leeches in the Medical Practice

Blood stasis in the head

Pooling, or slowing, of blood in the head may lead to cardiovascular diseases as well as other problems. Some of the symptoms include feeling a heavy weight in the head, pain in the eyes, sleeplessness, irritable/gloomy mood, loss of balance, dizziness, and blood rushes to the head when bending over. At times, the patient can feel a head rush and experience a flushed face while suffering from coldness in extremities and paling skin. A collection of these symptoms usually lead to a stroke.

If symptoms are moderate, the patient first needs to adjust his regiment by eating healthier, consuming smaller portions, reducing any intense physical activity, avoiding stress, getting more fresh air, and increasing blood circulation through light exercises such as walking. Cold compress, such as a towel soaked in cold water and applied to the head, may be helpful as well.

The patient may also massage his feet and submerge them in hot water. Afterwards, the patient should put on cotton socks, which were first soaked in water of about 60° F and then thoroughly wrung out. After that, dry woolen socks are placed over the cotton socks. This procedure is repeated several times a day, especially before bed to aid in the elimination of any contributing factors such as a cough or chest congestion. It is also beneficial to take infusions or drink herbal teas, designed to help in these situations.

If these methods do not help or the situation worsens to the point where the patient constantly experiences rushes of blood to the head, high blood pressure in the arteries, feels threatened with a stroke, then it is time to use leech therapy and apply leeches to the tailbone area (as further described in detail in Chapter 7). Local attachments, such as the ones behind the ear, can only help to reduce the plethora (*excess*) of blood in the head, but will not provide the full and lasting effect such as that of sessions focused on the entire organism, rather than just the affected area.

During blood stasis in the head, a patient may experience a nosebleed as a result of the organism's defense mechanism. This shouldn't alarm the patient though, because it may actually lead to an improved condition. *(Note: It is extremely rare to find cases where a nosebleed threatens a person's life.)*

It is not recommended to place the leech on the nasal septum (*the divider between the two nostrils*), except when the blood pressure in the head is caused by a viral infection, because placing a leech on the septum may draw even more blood to the head. However, when a person is carrying a deep infection along with high blood pressure in the head, a person may experience migraines, sleeplessness, and a flushed face. When a nosebleed occurs in this situation, it can lead to a temporary improvement and even help to reduce body temperature. If such an improvement is observed, then one should not wait and immediately apply leeches to the septum.

It is important to be able to estimate leech therapy's effect on the patient considering the factors of high blood pressure, anemia, or the weakening of the patient.

Blood stasis in the spine area

Pain in the spine as well as in the area of sciatic nerves have similar symptoms to blood stasis in the head and seldom occur independently of other symptoms. The pain is typically caused by the blood stasis and hyperemia (*increased flood flow to the tissues*) in the area. It is necessary to confirm that the cause of the pain is not the nerves themselves by checking with a neurologist to see if there may be underlying neurological (*nerve*) problems.

If after all hyperemia of the spinal cord and membrane is indeed the problem, you may place the leeches on the tailbone area instead of the spine to get the desired effect and relieve the plethora of blood.

Blood stasis in the chest area

Coughing up blood (*hemoptysis*) is usually a symptom of blood stasis in the chest area, although it should be duly noted that it can be caused by many other different things and may happen to people who do not have organic diseases of lungs and heart, to the young and even borderline healthy individuals.

Some doctors attribute this condition to angionecrosis (*deteriorating blood vessel walls*). And if it does not stop after employing regular methods of healing, then leech therapy may help. Although leech therapy stops the expectoration (*coughing up*) of blood, the patient should take on the responsibility to prevent a relapse. To do so, one needs to take immediate actions: overall strengthening of the organism, alleviating fatigue and anxiety, and following the recommendations of a specialist on angionecrosis.

One of the symptoms of tuberculosis is the expectoration of blood. If this persists, then one may apply leeches to the tailbone area. This should not only stop the expectorations but also make the patient feel better. *(Note: Treatment by leech therapy becomes ineffective when a cavity has developed in the lungs (from tuberculosis) causing the destruction of blood vessels and resulting in massive internal bleeding.)*

Hemoptysis alongside heart problems—mainly in the main veins—is usually accompanied by blood stasis in the liver and swellings (*edema*) of other organs. If it has not been possible to restore the full functions of the heart, then the use of leech therapy around the tailbone area is recommended.

Blood stasis in the stomach area

Most often, this condition is caused by poor blood circulation in the portal venous system (*main vein around the stomach area*), heart disease, liver disease, and weight problems. In these instances, it is recommended to apply leeches to the tailbone.

Those who suffer from an enlarged liver should not use leech therapy. These patients usually experience the vomiting of bile, a bitter taste in the mouth, jaundice, stool discoloration and dark brown urine. These patients need to look for individual methods of healing that may include medicinal herbs, homeopathic means, or other approaches specifically tailored to the individual's conditions.

Hemorrhoids

Hemorrhoids are caused by high blood pressure in the veins of the anus and are one of the most widespread diseases in all age groups. For most this condition is often the result of tension in the stomach (during constipation, pregnancy, etc.), while others are genetically predisposed to it.

Hemorrhoids can be internal and external, and range in size from a pea to a walnut. They typically are accompanied by a great deal of problems such as pain, swelling, inflammation, and bleeding. The patient may also be prone to thrombosis and the buildup of blood clots.

Often, one of first signs is rectal bleeding. In the beginning, one may notice traces of blood on the toilet paper, and later on the stool itself. At times, there can be a lot of bleeding without any visible signs (like knots). But even if the bleeding is seemingly insigificant, which can happen often, it can lead to anemia.

There are numerous benefits to using leech therapy as the choice of treatment. By placing leeches on the tailbone area one is able to simultaneously drain the affected area and also divert the blood flow, which, in turn, has a very strong healing effect. To reach this goal, it is recommended to use three to four leeches.

Unfortunately, even when faced with mild cases of hemorrhoids, doctors who know little about leech therapy are all too quick to recommend a complex procedure that may involve surgery. But these proposed methods are often ineffective and cannot guarantee that the hemorrhoids will not develop again later because they do not address the underlying problems in the circulatory system in the area.

Conditions suitable for leech therapy

Respiratory system:

> Bronchitis; pulmonary heart disease associated with chronic obstruction of the lungs and bronchial asthma; obesity hypoventilation syndrome (*also known as Pickwickian syndrome*); heavy pneumonia with difficulty breathing; arteries with thrombosis (in the lungs); tuberculosis accompanied by blood vomiting.

Urinary system:

> Pyelonephritis (*type of urinary tract infection*) with a hypertension syndrome; hypostases (*the settling of blood in relatively lower parts of an organ or the body due to impaired or absent circulation*); chronic nephritic syndrome (*kidney disorder*); cystitis (*urinary bladder inflammation*).

Musculoskeletal system:

> Radiculitis (*pain associated with the nerves stemming out from the spine, usually due to inflammation*); arthritises.

Digestive system:

> Hemorrhoids; pancreatitis; hemostasis (blood stasis) in the liver, cirrhosis; cholecystitis (*inflammation of the gallbladder*) and other chronic inflammations in the abdominal cavity.

Cardiovascular system:

Asystole; Raynaud's disease; high blood pressure; lymphostasis (*stoppage of lymph flow*); ischemic heart trouble; stenocardia; pre heart attack symptoms; heart attack (heart spasms, blood clots); inflamed blood vessels; poor blood circulation; heart muscles diseases; obliterative arterial disease; obliterative thromboangiitis; trophic ulcer (of veins and arteries).

Obstetrics (female reproductive system) and gynecology:

Inflammatory conditions; complications during the postnatal period; problems with mammary glands (and forms of mastitis); a thrombophlebitis (*inflammation of a vein caused by a blood clot*) of the pelvic region; toxicosis during pregnancy; menopause.

Dermatology (skin):

Scleroderma; eczema; lupus; toxidermia; chronic form of dermatitis; psoriasis; erysipelatous inflammation of the skin. (You may forgo surgery and treat these conditions with leech therapy by placing leeches on the affected area or conducting whole organism treatments.)

Otolaryngology (nose, throat, ears):

Acute and chronic pain of the acoustic (*auditory*) nerve; constant noise in the ears; acute and chronic otitis (*inflammation/infection of the ear*); auditory canal infection (that penetrates inside); antritis; inflammation of frontal sinuses; inflammation of cells in the ethmoid bone.

Ophthalmology (eyes):

Leech therapy may also be used during iritis; burst blood vessels in the eyes; macular retinal dystrophy; inflammation of blood vessels in the eye; and glaucoma. It has been established that even when leeches are attached to one side of the face, the other side reacts as well helping the second eye inflicted with glaucoma. In any case, the treatment should be tailored for each individual. Clinically, it has been shown that the pressure is relieved within three hours after the treatment and the relief is further amplified by the secretion of inner eye fluids. Some doctors believe that using leech therapy during advanced stages of glaucoma is not advisable because if leech therapy is not successful, then using other methods and/or even having surgery following leech attachments may lead to hyphema (*bleeding in the front area of the eye*).

Neuropathology:

Various diseases of the central nervous system—like atherosclerosis and thrombosis of the vessels in the brain—may hinder the blood circulation in the head and contribute to loss of consciousness, stroke, loss of hearing, stagnation of blood, paralysis, bruising, concussion, nerve damage, and migraines. When leech therapy is used in the case of a concussion (when there is no fracture of the skull), the symptoms almost disappear. Thus, leech therapy, alongside conventional medical methods, may have a bright future as a treatment of nerve diseases, as well as a preventive measure against complications.

Stomatology:

Leeches can be used in combination with other approaches to treat oral diseases including gingivitis, periodontitis, acute and chronic canker sores, and glossodynia (*tongue pain*).

Surgery:

Leech therapy may be a powerful tool in postoperative maintenance and can be used to address possible problems such as infiltration, postoperative blood clots, and the deficiency of blood flow in the veins after microsurgery. It may help after surgery and treatment following a gunshot wound (that may require very detailed work on torn body tissues). It may also help after reconstructive surgery, pathological breakdowns of the blood system in the area such as varicose veins, various forms of thrombophlebitis, and lymphostasis of lower extremities.

Searching for answers

The forms of pathology, specified above, can help us to develop the general guidelines for leech therapy aimed at the restoration of homeostasis of the body. Although, in the past, it was believed that leech treatments only benefited the patient by just the mechanical action of bleeding, today, through medical research we know that leech treatments not only act to help the area of application, but also have an impact on the entire organism of the patient.

Remember, due to the body's strong responses to leech therapy during complex diseases, it is very important to conduct more research to exactly pinpoint all of the benefits of leeches on human health.

7

Step by Step Instructions

Attachment zones and points

Doctors and healers usually follow the signs that lead them to the right method of treatment. And the signs that lead to leech therapy are no different because this method's efficiency is substantially related to the specialist's ability to understand the patient's condition and tailor a treatment to a particular disease.

It is important to understand that the diagnosis *per se* is not the most important part of this process. But what is more important is the right treatment of symptoms and effects of the disease (like lymphostasis, blood stasis in organs and tissues, thrombosis in arteries or veins, or damaged nutritional processes of the cells).

Today, leech therapy is experiencing a re-birth in the medical field and some of the most frequently asked questions are: where to place the leeches, in what area on the body, and at what exact points?

For the most part, there are no uniform zones. But the knowledge of Eastern medicine provides us with general points on the body that correspond to a deeper connection to the internal organs. These guidelines allow most specialists to design a system of placement that corresponds to different diseases. Since it is extremely important to be able to accurately identify these points on the body, this book includes several images to help you find these places.

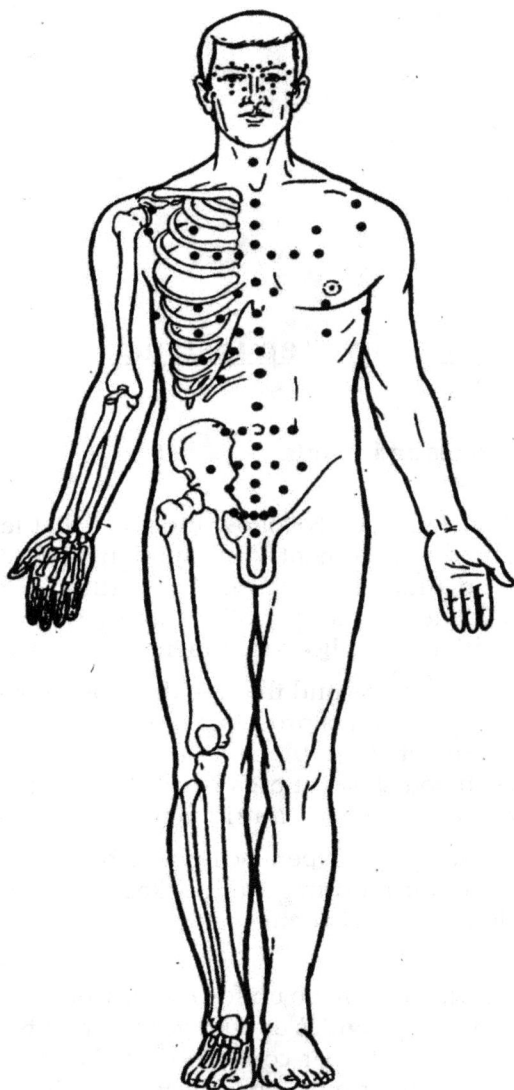

General Attachment Points - Front

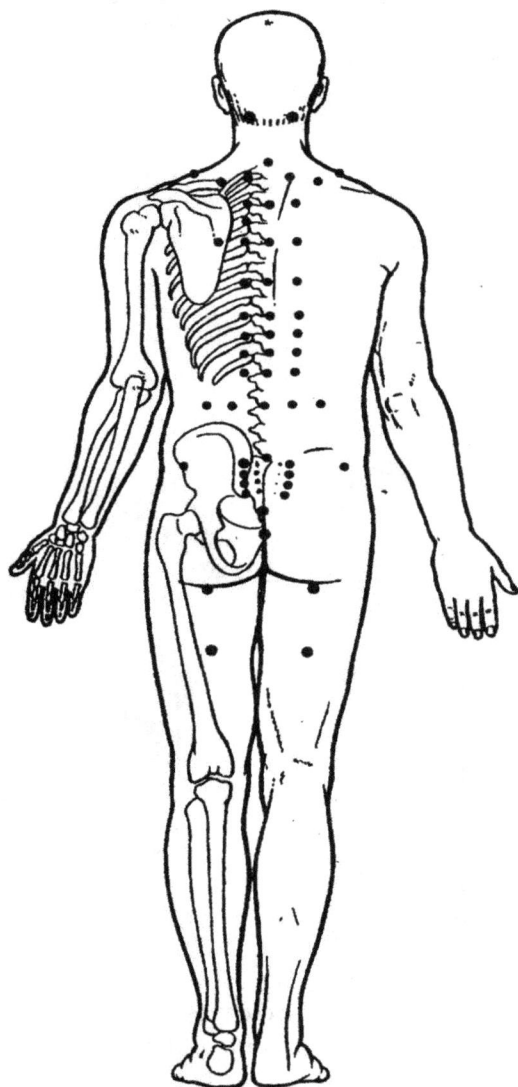

General Attachment Points - Rear

Keep in mind that with proper knowledge and your doctor's permission, you may be able to conduct leech therapy in household conditions. Without the supervision of your doctor or therapist, however, you have to act in strict accordance with their advice at all times. Otherwise, you risk inflicting a great harm on yourself and others.

Chest pain

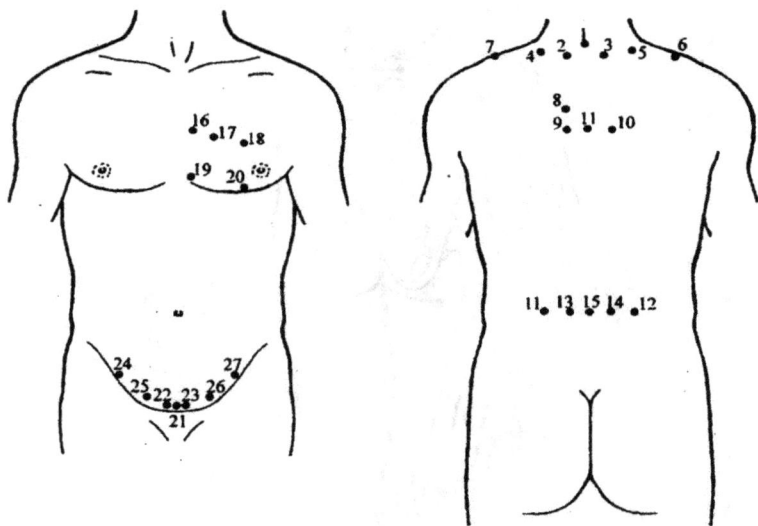

This type of pain is typically located around the heart and may vary in length and intensity: pricking, aching, piercing, sharp, momentary, lasting hours and even days (as though there is a stone lying on your heart). The pain is usually felt in the left part of the chest and may stretch as far as the left hand and back. Chest pains are often accompanied by various symptoms including: a strong connection with pain of the spine around the neck and chest level, diseases of the common bile duct, and hormonal imbalance. Oftentimes, physical activity has no effect on the pain, and neither does consumption of nitrates or other medications commonly used to prevent and relieve chest pain.

Attachment Zones:

Zone 1
Top of the spine area
Points 1, 2, 3
Points 2 and 3 are 2 to 4 centimeters away from the
center Point 1, which is located underneath C7, the
bottom cervical vertebrae.

Zone 2
Area of the shoulders
Points 4, 5, 6, 7
Points 4, 5, 6, and 7 are located in the middle of the
left and right shoulders

Zone 3
Area of the heart
Points 16, 17, 18, 19, 20
Point 16 is underneath the third rib near the sternum.
Points 17 and 18 are 1 to 2 inch intervals from Point 16.
Point 19 is on the edge of the chest right below the
fifth rib and Point 20 is on the middle bottom edge
of the chest.

Zone 4
Area between the shoulder blades
Points 8, 9, 10, 11
Point 11 is on T5-6, the fifth or sixth thoracic vertebrae.
Points 9 and 10 are 1 to 2 inches to the right and left.
Point 8 is on the level of T4-5.

Zone 5
Area of the lower back
Points 11, 12, 13, 14, 15
Point 15 is located at L2-3, second or third lumbar
vertebrae. Points 11, 12, 13, and 14 are spaced from the
center point at 1 to 2 inches intervals.

Zone 6
Area of the pelvis
Points 21-27
Points 21, 22, 23, 24, 25, 26, and 27 are spread in a semi circle on the lower abdomen starting at the center over the pubis (*pubic bone*).

Procedure Overview:

When there is nerve pain and pain in the spine, use Zones 1, 2, 3 and 4. In the case of hormonal imbalance, use Zones 3, 4, 5, and 6.

Quantity of attachments:

Use 3 to 4 per session. When including Zones 3 and 4, use 4 to 8 leeches per course.

Quantity of sessions:

First 3 to 4 sessions should be conducted every other day using different zones, followed by additional 4 sessions 2 times a week. To solidify the effects of the entire course, follow-up with 2 to 3 sessions with a longer wait time in between. For aches and pains that have continued for a long time, make sure to include 2 to 3 sessions concentrating on Zone 3.

Combination healing:

While leech therapy can be the main treatment, for additional healing benefits, drink infusions and teas, such as hawthorn, intended for cardiovascular health.

Stenocardia (*angina*)

Stenocardia results in heart problems and pain caused by deterioration in blood circulation and lack of oxygen in the heart (*ischemia*). The main symptom of stenocardia is chest pressure sensation that usually increases during physical activities.

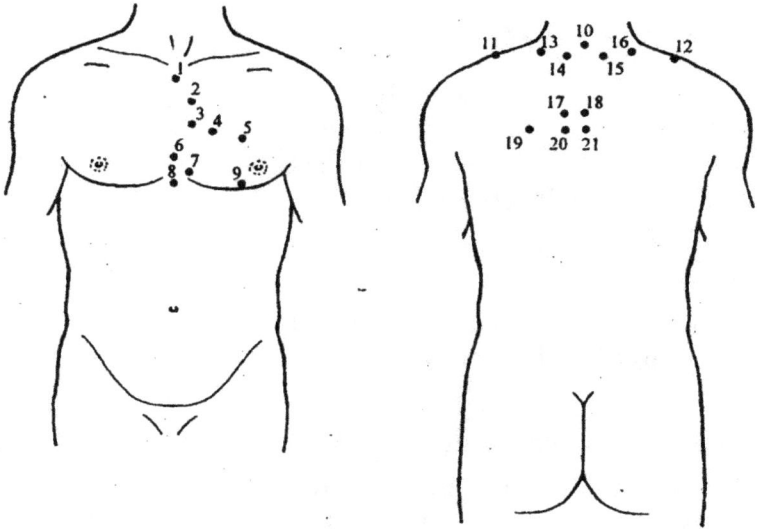

Attachment Zones:

Zone 1
Area around the heart
Points 3, 4, 5, 7, 9
Point 3 is located right below the third rib from the top, on the edge of the chest. Points 4 and 5 are at 1 to 2 inch intervals from Point 3. Point 7 is on the bottom corner edge of the chest, right below the fifth rib. Point 9 is on the bottom middle edge of the chest.

Zone 2
Area between the shoulder blades
Points 17, 18, 19, 20 21
Point 18 is on the level of T4-5, the fourth or fifth thoracic vertebrae. Point 21 is on T5-6, the fifth or sixth thoracic vertebrae. Points 17, 19, 20 are on the same levels at 1 to 2 inch intervals.

(cont.)

Zone 3
Area around the sternum
Points 1, 6, 8
All points are on the same line as the sternum. Point 8 is located on the tip of the xiphoid process with Point 6 slightly above that on the same level as the bottom ribs. Point 1 is located over the manubrium.

Procedure Overview:

The first 2 to 3 sessions should be done over Zone 1. Afterwards, other zones should be included as well.

Quantity of attachments:

Each session should have an increased number of leeches ranging from 2-6. Depending on the severity of your condition, this number could be as high as 10 leeches per session. In this particular instance, a specialist should remove the leeches when they have begun to freely consume the blood (and long before they fall off on their own).

Quantify of sessions:

First 3 to 5 sessions should be conducted daily until the pain subsides considerably. Continue with 3 sessions every other day with 3 to 4 sessions weekly. The entire course of treatment is 10 sessions. Depending on the status of the patient the course may be repeated after 2 to 4 weeks.

Healing combinations:

Although leech therapy can be the main treatment, you may also supplement it with medicinal herbs intended for cardiovascular health for a duration of 3 months.

Hypertension (*high blood pressure*)

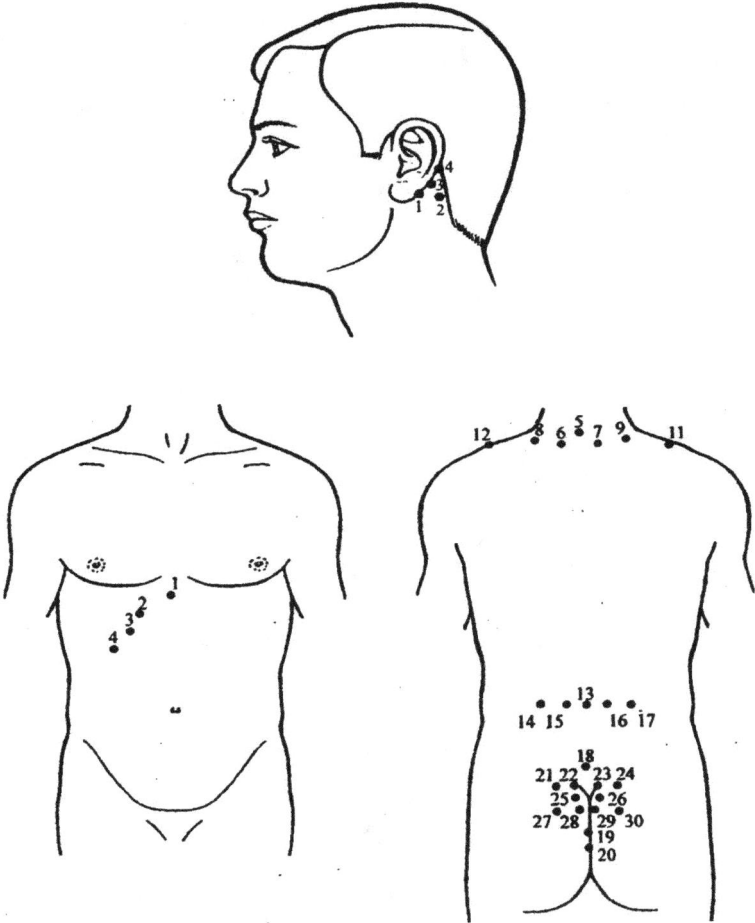

The main symptom is the high blood pressure in the arteries. This could be the result of stress, hormonal imbalance, kidney disease, diet, lifestyle, etc. but most often there are numerous contributing factors to this condition. Therefore, to design the most successful treatment plan one needs to figure out all the contributing factors first.

Leech therapy is a great choice of treatment in mild or strong cases. In the case of hypertension, leech therapy can be especially useful during the most difficult times when there is a sudden jump in the blood pressure, which may be quite dangerous and could increase the chance of a stroke.

Attachment Zones:

Zone 1
Area around the ear
Points 1, 2, 3, 4
Points 1, 2, 3, and 4 are all retro auricular (*behind the ear*) spots located right near the edge of the helix.

Zone 2
Area around the tailbone
Points 19-30
Points 19 and 20 are near the tip of the tailbone. Points 21-30 are located around the sacrum.

Zone 3
Area of the lower neck
Points 5, 6, 7
Point 5 is located on C7, the bottom cervical vertebrae. Points 6 and 7 are located 1 to 2 inches from Point 5.

Zone 4
Area of the shoulders
Points 8, 9, 11, 12
Points 8, 9, 11, and 12 are located on the middle parts of the shoulders.

Zone 5
Area of the lower back
Points 13, 14, 15, 16, 17
Point 13 is located at L2-3, second or third lumbar vertebrae. Points 14, 15, 16, and 17 are located at 1 to 2 inch intervals from the center Point 13.

Zone 6
Liver area
Points 1, 2, 3, 4
Points start at the highest point right below the bottom
right rib and go down at intervals of 1 to 2 inches.

Procedure Overview:

Applying leech therapy to treat hypertension is an art
in itself. The number of leeches, the points of placement,
the intensity of treatments and other factors should be
tailored to the individual's state of health as well as all
other factors that are causing this condition. But, at the
very least, leech therapy has the potential to reduce
many of the uncomfortable symptoms of hypertension.

At the time of treatment, Zones 3 and 4 are used in
combination with Zone 2 during the same sessions. This
approach is especially useful when a patient experiences
symptoms of vegetative-vascular dystonia including
dizziness, blood rush, and sweating. In addition, it
could be very effective in treating emotional imbalance,
such as recurring anger or hysterical outbursts.

Zone 2 is the most important in hypertension treatment.
If there is also a developing disease in the kidneys, it is
important to include Zone 5 while focusing on the side
of the body with the troubled kidney.

When hypertension emergency strikes, it can be a
handful. Leech therapy's success during this emergency
situation gives it an advantage over medicine that leads
to insignificant or temporary results. It is the leech
therapy's ability to treat the entire body that makes
is so effective.

In the beginning of the treatment, concentrate on
Zone 2 first. Then move to Zone 6, which is then
followed by Zone 1.

*(Caution: On rare occasions, depending on the severity
of the condition, local applications may lead to a reverse
effect and actually draw blood to the veins instead of the
other way around.)*

Quantity of attachments:

During a hypertensive emergency, use up to 4 leeches per session. When the blood pressure decreases, the number of leeches should be decreased as well.

Quantity of sessions:

In extreme cases, sessions can be conducted daily. When the blood pressure decreases, the number of sessions can be reduced to 1 to 2 times a week. Course of healing is 7 to 9 sessions.

Healing combinations:

Leech therapy should be used in combination with healthy natural foods, relaxation therapy, and herbal medicine. Fasting may help as well.

Heart failure

Heart failure is the inability of the heart to supply sufficient blood flow to meet the body's needs. Common causes are myocardial infarction and forms of ischemic heart disease, cardiomyopathy, high blood pressure, valvular heart disease, and chronic lung diseases. Most often heart failure is caused by a combination of ischemic heart disease and hypertensive disease. Symptoms include shortness of breath, coughing, pneumonia, cardiac asthma, and swelling of the lungs and other places.

Attachment Zones:

Zone 1
Area around the heart
Points 3, 4, 5, 7, 8
Point 3, 4, and 5 are around the heart area right under the third rib. Point 8 is under the fifth rib on the bottom center of the left chest muscle. Point 7 is under the fifth rib on the bottom right corner of the left chest muscle.

Zone 2
Area around the sternum
Points 1, 2, 6
Point 1 and 2 are located on the manubrium sterni, which is the broad upper part of the sternum and is on the level with the first two ribs. Point 6 is on the level of the fifth rib.

Zone 3
Area around the sacrum and the tailbone
Points 16-26
Point 17 and 18 are located on the bottom tip of the tailbone. Points 16 and 19-26 are outlining the sacrum.

Zone 4
Area of the liver
Points 9-15
The bottom row of Points 9-15 are positioned right below the rib cage, while the rest are moving up towards the liver area.

Procedure Overview:

People with heart failure often require a lengthy treatment. If heart failure develops with a plethora of blood in the area, then the liver increases in size. In this situation, the patient experiences crepitation in the lungs (*wheezing*) and thus, the leeches are left on for maximum amount of time until they fall off on their own.

During functional deterioration (*decompensation*), the zones of the liver and the tailbone become more important.

For improvement of the heart muscle function, the zones around the heart have the best effect.

Quantity of attachments:

4 to 6 per session. If the condition improves significantly, then the number of leeches should be decreased to 3 or 4 per session for the rest of the treatment.

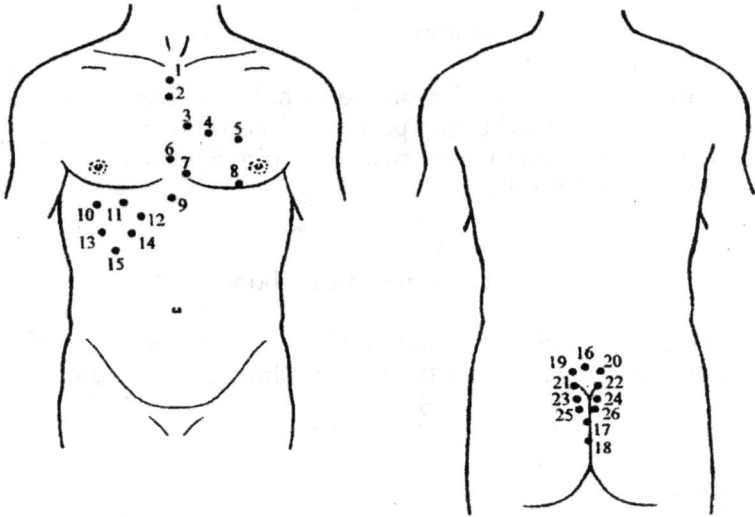

Quantity of attachments:

4 to 6 per session. If the condition improves significantly, then the number of leeches should be decreased to 3 or 4 per session for the rest of the treatment.

Quantity of sessions:

Sessions should be administered no more than 1 to 2 times a week. The usual course of treatment is 7 to 12 sessions, with special attention paid to the zones that are affected the most.

Healing combinations:

Although leech therapy may be the main treatment, it is essential to combine it with a healthy diet and herbal tea designed for cardiovascular health and increased urination (*diuretic*). It is also beneficial to cleanse the stomach and the liver.

Bronchitis

Acute and chronic bronchitis are inflammatory conditions in the bronchial tubes. Acute bronchitis is less severe and is usually caused by viruses and certain bacteria.

Chronic bronchitis is frequently a reaction to the environment and develops over time to due to cigarette smoke, exposure to chemicals and air pollution among many others. Bronchitis is most often an allergic reaction of the organism. It also weakens the immune system, especially that of the elderly.

The main symptom is coughing, which increases with cold and humid weather. When suffering from bronchitis, one may cough up mucous, which varies in characteristics and quantity. When producing very thick mucus, due to acute or chronic bronchitis, leech therapy can be very effective. In other cases, leech therapy is used in combination with other treatments by strengthening the immune system, improving the metabolism and decreasing venous plethora.

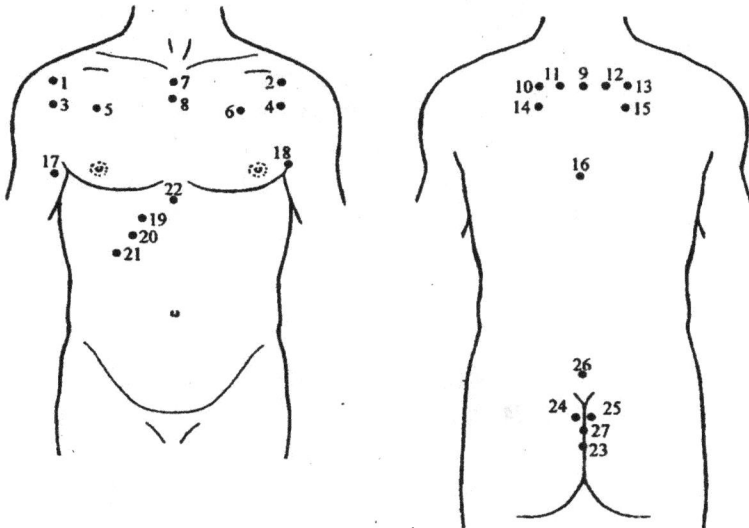

Attachment Zones:

Zone 1
Area of the lungs
Points 1, 2, 3, 4, 5, 6, 7, 8
Points 1, 2, 3, and 4 are on the level of the first and
second ribs, on the outside of the chest over the deltoids.
Symmetrically place Points 5 and 6 by starting near the
sternum underneath the second rib and moving out
parallel to the collarbone. Points 7 and 8 are located on
the broad upper part of the sternum (*manubrium sterni*).

Zone 2
Area of the spleen
Points 17 and 18
Points 17 and 18 are located symmetrically on the same
level on both sides of the body about 2 to 3 inches below
the top of the arc of the armpit.

Zone 3
Area between the shoulder blades
Points 9, 10, 11, 12, 13, 14, 15, 16
Point 9 is located on T3-4, the third or fourth thoracic
vertebrae. Points 10, 11, 12, and 13 are on the same level
and are located at 1 to 2 inch intervals. Points 14 and
15 are located about one inch below Points 10 and 13,
respectively. Point 16 is in the middle of the back on the
level with the bottom tips of the shoulder blades.

Zone 4
Area around the sacrum and the tailbone
Points 23, 24, 25, 26, 27
Points 23 and 27 are located on the bottom tip of the
tailbone. Points 24, 25, and 26 are outlining the sacrum.

Zone 5
Area around the liver
Points 19, 20, 21, 22

Points 19, 20, and 21 are right below the right bottom rib. Point 22 is located on the bottom tip of the sternum (*xiphoid process*).

Procedure Overview:

Sessions are consistently done in Zones 1, 2, and 3. The points between the shoulder blades are the most significant. Leeches are left attached until they fall off on their own. Points 3 & 4 and 11 & 12 are usually used in pairs; the others are usually placed on the affected side. Zones 4 and 5 are important to use when there is blood stasis in the lungs or pneumonia.

Quantity of attachments:

During the first few sessions, use 2 to 3 leeches. Then, gradually increase up to 5 to 7.

Quantity of sessions:

3 to 4 sessions every other day, then, twice a week. Course of treatment consists of 7 to 8 sessions.

Combination healing:

Leech therapy is a complimentary treatment. It works well when used in combination with compresses, breathing therapy, and herbal medicine. Massage is also recommended.

Asthma

Asthma is an inflammation of bronchial tubes that causes an obstruction of the airways. The symptoms include shortness of breath, coughing, tightness in the chest, development of mucous and wheezing. It may develop alongside excess of blood (*plethora*) in the area of the chest, abdominal cavity, and pelvic cavity. Careful consideration of all the details is important for setting up the right treatment strategy for the individual.

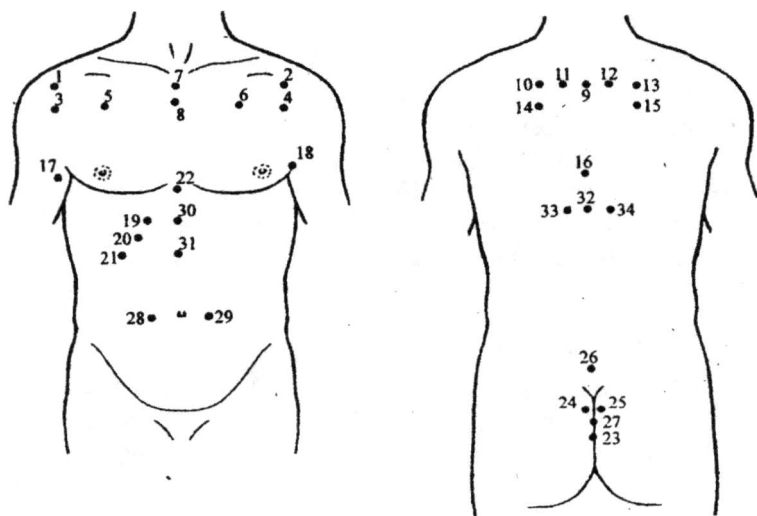

Attachment Zones:

Zone 1
Area of the lungs
Points 1-8
Points 1, 2, 3, and 4 are on the level with the first and second rib. Points 5 and 6 are symmetrical and are located under the second rib. Points 7 and 8 are located on the broad upper part of the sternum (*manubrium sterni*).

Zone 2
Area of the arm pits
Points 17 and 18 are located symmetrically on the same level on both sides of the body about 2 to 3 inches below the top of the arc of the armpit.

Zone 3
Area between the shoulder blades
Points 9, 10, 11, 12, 13, 14, 15, 16
Point 9 is located on T3-4, the third or fourth thoracic
vertebrae. Points 10, 11, 12, and 13 are on the same level
and are located at 1 to 2 inch intervals. Points 14 and
15 are located about one inch below Points 10 and 13,
respectively. Point 16 is in the middle of the back on the
level with the bottom tips of the shoulder blades.

Zone 4
Areas around the sacrum and the tailbone
Points 23, 24, 25, 26, 27
Points 23 and 27 are located on the bottom tip of the
tailbone. Points 24, 25, and 26 are outlining the sacrum.

Zone 5
Area around the liver
Points 19, 20, 21, 22
Points 19, 20, and 21 are right below the right bottom
rib. Point 22 is located on the bottom part of the sternum
(*xiphoid process*).

Zone 6
Area of the stomach
Points 28, 29, 30, 31
Points 28 and 29 are symmetric. They are on the level
with the belly button and are about 1 to 2 inches from
it. Points 30 and 31 are right down the middle over the
stomach (and usually these points are painful to touch).

Zone 7
Area between the shoulder blades
Points 32, 33, 34
Point 32 is on the center of the body on the level
with T9-10, the ninth or tenth thoracic vertebrae.
Points 33 and 34 are 1 to 2 inches away from
Point 32 and on the same level.

Procedure Overview:

Creating an effective therapy schedule for asthma is an artful display of the doctor's knowledge and experience. Besides including Zones 1, 2 and 3, follow any signs of hyperemia (*excess of blood flow to a particular tissue or organ*) to include other ones. If it shows up mainly in the chest cavity organs, use Zones 1, 2, 3, and 4. If it shows up in the abdominal cavity organs, add Zones 5, 6, and 7. If it shows up mainly in the organs of the pelvic cavity, add Zone 4 and use a larger quantity of attachments per session.

Quantity of attachments:

As a rule, it is not good to rush in with a large quantity of leeches. Start with as little as 2 per session. In rare cases it may be 6 to 8 per session. But usually it is 3 or 4. The quantity of leeches should depend on the severity of the condition and the inteded length of treatment.

Quantity of sessions:

In the beginning, the first 4 sessions are administered twice a week. Then, shift to just one time a week with up to 7 to 8 sessions for the entire course. Repeat 3 times with 2 to 4 week breaks between courses.

Combination healing:

Leech therapy is a very effective means of healing especially in the presence of venous plethora or hyperemia. However, it is necessary to supplement leech therapy with hot compresses to the chest, breathing exercises, healthy dieting, cleansing of the organs, and herbal medicine. Also, fasting yields great results (but should never be done during the same time as leech therapy).

Gastritis

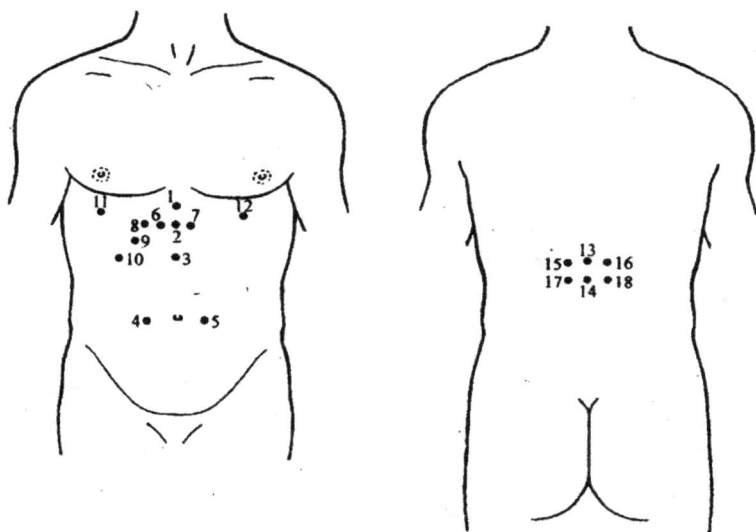

Gastritis is an inflammation of the stomach lining. It has many possible causes and some doctors do not consider it as an individual disease but in combination with other digestion problems. It is caused by a number of reasons: not eating a healthy diet, accumulation of waste products in the body and psychological overload (like stress). As a result, some ability of the organs to function is damaged including the stomach, pancreas, and small and large intestines. In particular, the glands of the digestive tracts suffer. Symptoms include loss of appetite, feeling bloated, rumbling, pain in the stomach, and irregular bowel movements. Usually, this leads to damage in the liver and gall bladder, and further complications in digesting food which may result in a slower metabolism.

Attachment Zones:

Zone 1
Area of the stomach
Points 2, 3, 4, 5, 6, 7
Points 4 and 5 are symmetrical points on the level with

the belly button. Points 2 and 3 are in the middle over the stomach and are usually the points of pain. Points 6 and 7 are on same level as Point 2 and are 1 to 2 inches away.

Zone 2
Area of the spine
Points 13-18
Point 13 is located on T11-12, the eleventh or twelfth thoracic vertebrae. Point 14 is located on T12-L1, the twelfth thoracic vertebrae or the first lumbar vertebrae. Points 15-18 are on the same level, respectively, about 1 to 2 inches from the center points, 13 and 14.

Zone 3
Area of the liver
Points 1, 8, 9, 10, 11, 12
Points 8, 9 and 10 are right underneath the right bottom rib. Points 11 and 12 are underneath the sixth rib. Point 1 is located on the xiphoid process, which is the bottom part of the sternum.

Procedure Overview:

Use the zones indicated above.

Quantity of attachments:

2 to 3 per session. Do not use more than 2 attachments per zone. Points 4 & 5, 1 & 2, 15 & 16, 17 & 18 are strong healing pairs.

Quantity of sessions:

The first two sessions are conducted 3 days apart, then sessions are held once a week. Course of healing consists of 7 sessions.

Combination healing:

The results of leech therapy could be greatly improved if it is administered after fasting for three days. After the treatment, follow with a healthy diet, hydrotherapy (up to 3 months), and herbal medicine.

Chronic hepatitis and cirrhosis

Chronic hepatitis and cirrhosis (*scarring of the liver*) diseases often develop following an infectious jaundice. It could also be the result of chemicals exposure, alcohol abuse, or dysfunctional outflow of bile. Both conditions results in deterioration of liver cells. In these cases, leech therapy is absolutely necessary, and it is more effective if started in the early stages of the disease.

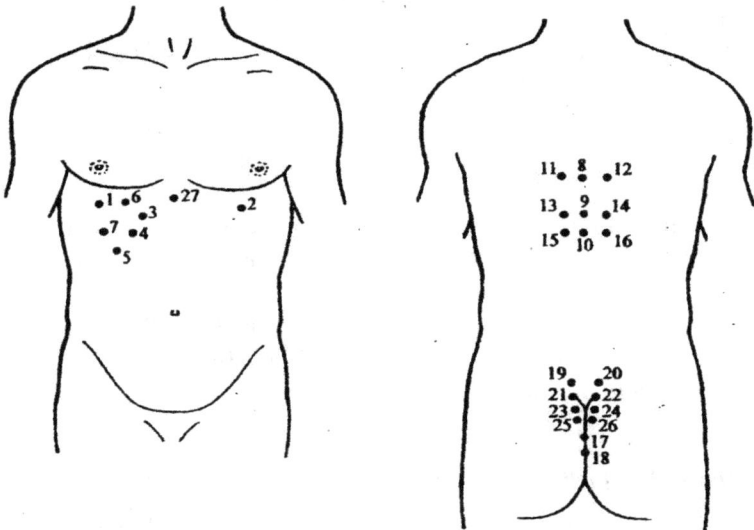

Attachment Zones:

Zone 1
Area of the liver
Points 1, 2, 3, 4, 5, 6, 7, 27
Points 3, 4 and 5 are right underneath the right bottom
rib. Points 6 and 7 are over the liver. Points 1 and 2 are
underneath the sixth rib. Point 27 is located on the tip
of the xiphoid process, which is the bottom part of
the sternum.

Zone 2
Area of the spine
Points 8, 9, 10, 11, 12, 13, 14, 15, 16
Point 8 is located on T7-8, the seventh or eighth thoracic
vertebrae. Point 9 is located on T8-9, the eighth or ninth
thoracic vertebrae. Point 10 is located on T9-10, the ninth
or tenth thoracic vertebrae. Points 11-16 are respectively
1 to 2 inches away from the center points.

Zone 3
Area around the sacrum and the tailbone
Points 17, 18, 19-26
Points 17 and 18 are located on the bottom tip of the
tailbone. Points 19-26 are outlining the sacrum.

Procedure Overview:

Because a large number of leeches (4 to 8) is necessary
per session, they should be removed early.
Zone 1 is the most important.
Zone 3 becomes more important during signs of
functional deterioration, such as ascites (*which is an
accumulation of fluids in the abdomen*).

Quantity of attachments:

4 to 8 per session. Since the course of treatment is long,
it is necessary to increase intake of iron through iron-

rich foods (though not red meat) and supplements, while periodically testing its level in the blood.

Quantity of sessions:

Sessions are held twice a week at first and then once a week until the total number of sessions reaches 12. This course may be repeated after 30 to 45 days.

Combination healing:

Although leech therapy can be the main treatment, a greater effect could be achieved by combining it with an improved diet and herbal supplements.

Ulcer of the stomach and duodenum

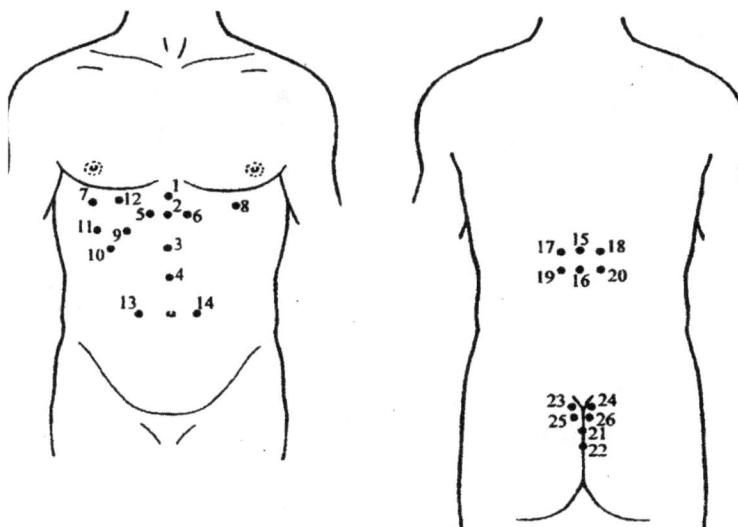

This type of ulcer is an inflammation usually caused by the weakening of the stomach wall. Leech therapy can be the primary treatment, especially when there are signs of inflammation.

In other cases it may serve as a supplementary treatment by accelerating the healing process. Leech therapy becomes critical to use in a timely manner over the affected area if the duodenum begins to show signs of cicatricial deformations (*scarring*).

Attachment Zones:

Zone 1
Area of the stomach
Points 1, 2, 3, 4, 5, 6,
Points 2, 3, and 4 are placed down the center on the belly, which is usually the area of pain. And Point 1 is located on the xiphoid process, which is the bottom part of the sternum. Points 5 and 6 are on the same level as Point 2 at 1 to 2 inch intervals.

Zone 2
Area of the spine
Points 15, 16, 17, 18, 19, 20
Point 15 is located on T11-12, the eleventh or twelfth thoracic vertebrae. Point 16 is located on T12-L1, the twelfth thoracic vertebrae or the first lumbar vertebrae. Points 17-20 are on the same level, respectively, about 1 to 2 inches from the center Points 15 and 16.

Zone 3
Area of the liver
Points 7, 8, 9, 10, 11, 12
Points 9 and 10 are right underneath the right bottom rib. Points 11 and 12 are over the liver. Points 7 and 8 are underneath the sixth rib.

Zone 4
Area of the belly
Points 13 and 14
Points 13 and 14 are on the same level as the belly button about two inches on either side.

Zone 5
Area around the sacrum and the tailbone
Points 21, 22, 23-26

Points 21 and 22 are located on the bottom tip of the tailbone. Points 23-26 are outlining the sacrum.

Procedure Overview:

When there are signs of hyperemia (*excess of blood*) around the stomach area, it is beneficial to alternate between Zones 1 and 3, and 2 and 5. The quantity of leeches should be slightly more in Zones 3 and 4.
If the goal of leech therapy is to accelerate the healing process, then use at least two leeches per session on Zones 1 and 2.

Quantity of attachments:

Zones 1, 2, and 4, use 2 to 3 per session. Zones 3 and 5, use 3 to 5 per session. During inflammations, use up to 5 to 6 per session.

Quantity of sessions:

The first few sessions are conducted every other day and then twice a week. The duration of the course is determined by the patient's reaction to the treatment.

Combination healing:

It is necessary to combine leech therapy with herbal medicine and relaxation therapy while maintaining a healthy diet and consuming fresh juices along with biologically-active products.

Chronic constipation

Constipation can be brought on by many factors, some of which include poor diet, not enough exercise, and stress. About one-third of the population suffers from constipation at some point. (*Note: People frequently suffer from constipation and hemorrhoids simultaneously.*)

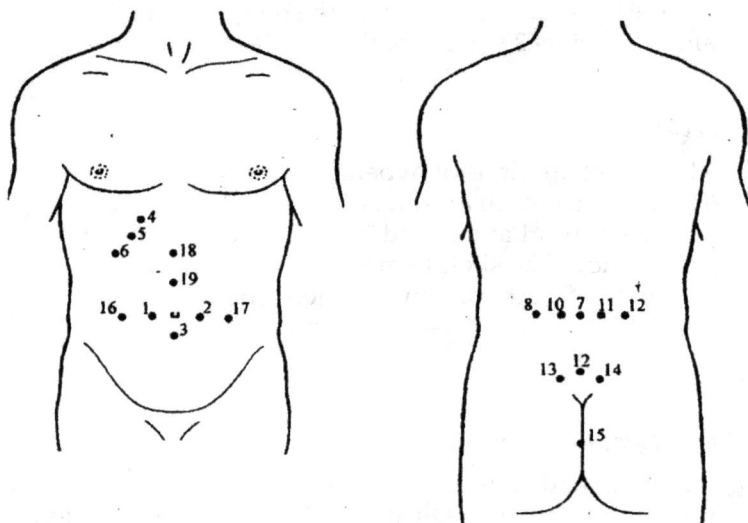

Attachment Zones:

Zone 1
Area of the midsection
Points 1, 2, 3, 16, 17, 18
Points 1, 2, 16 and 17 are symmetrically located at 1 to 2 inch intervals from each other starting with the belly button as the center. Points 18 and 19 are down the middle. Point 3 is located 2 to 3 inches below the belly button.

Zone 2
Area of the lower back
Points 7, 8, 10, 11, 12
Point 7 is located on L1-L2, the first or second lumbar vertebrae. Points 8, 10, 11, and 12 are located on the same level at 1 to 2 inch intervals from the center Point 7.

Zone 3
Area of the tailbone
Points 12, 13, 14, 15

Point 15 is located on the bottom tip of the tailbone.
Points 12, 13 and 14 are outlining the sacrum.

Zone 4
Area of the liver
Points 4, 5, 6
Points 4, 5 and 6 are right underneath the right
bottom rib.

Procedure Overview:

Leech therapy is a supplementary treatment for
constipation. However, it is absolutely necessary
when there is plethora (*excess*) of blood in the veins of
the abdominal cavity, when a person is old, or when
hemorrhoids are present.

Quantity of attachments:

3 to 5 per session

Quantity of sessions:

Sessions are held every other day and then
twice a week.

Combination healing:

Leech therapy should be accompanied by intestinal
cleansing (with enough fiber), restoration of microflora
of intestines, stomach massages and herbal medicine.

Chronic pancreatitis

Chronic pancreatitis is a disease that is widespread throughout
the population. It affects the stomach's functions causing pain
in the area as well as an inability to properly digest and absorb

food. Leech therapy has shown to be an effective treatment for this disease, especially in the presence of blood stasis in the abdominal cavity.

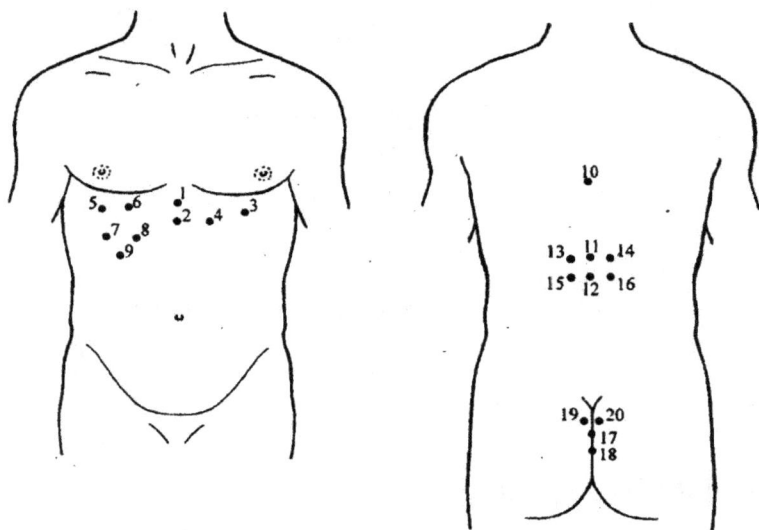

Attachment Zones:

Zone 1
Top of the stomach area
Points 1, 2, 3, 4
Points 1 and 2 are right down the middle and usually over an area of pain. Points 3 and 4 are usually the most effective because they are placed over the most painful area, the top left area of the stomach.

Zone 2
Area of the spine
Points 10-16
Point 10 is located on T7-8, the seventh or eighth thoracic vertebrae. Point 11 is located on T11-12, the eleventh or twelfth thoracic vertebrae. Point 12 is located on T12-L1, the twelfth thoracic vertebrae or the first lumbar vertebrae. Points 13-16 are on the same level, respectively, about 1 to 2 inches from the center Points 11 and 12.

Zone 3
Area of the liver
Points 5, 6, 7, 8, 9
Points 5-9 are located under the bottom rib
and over the liver.

Zone 4
Area of the tailbone
Points 17, 18, 19, 20
Points 17 and 18 are located on the bottom tip of the
tailbone. Points 19 and 20 are outlining the sacrum.

Procedure Overview:

Usually it is necessary to alternate among the points
in Zone 1 and 2 between sessions. To achieve better
results, it is important to identify those points where
most of the pain is located. Use the points in Zones 3
and 4 when there is excess blood in the veins of
the abdominal cavity.

Quantity of attachments:

3 to 5 per session

Quantity of sessions:

Use 3 leeches per session every other day and then
up to 7 to 9 leeches twice a week for the duration of
the healing process.

Combination healing:

Pancreatitis is usually not an isolated disease and the
treatment should aim to restore the entire digestive
system. Thus, it is also recommended to try other means
of treating the organs of the abdominal cavity: cleansing
the organism, a healthy diet, herbal medicine, and
breathing exercises.

Allergies

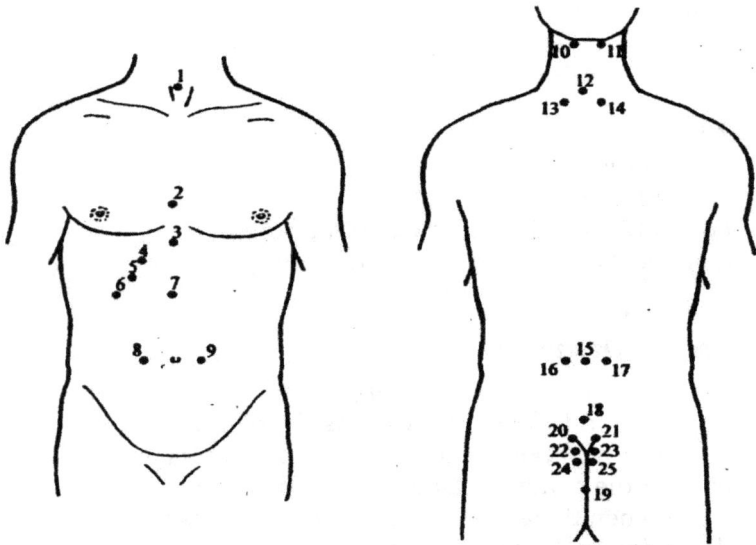

An allergy is an organism's response when an immune system overreacts to an external substance. There is a wide range of allergies, anywhere from airborne substances (asthma), to food, and medicine (to name a few). The cause is typically either an environmental factor or a genetic factor. Allergies result in microcirculation and lymphatic malfunctions in the veins and venous systems. Usually the skin or the mucous membrane is affected in the process.

Attachment Zones

Zone 1
Area of the neck
Points 1, 10, 11, 12, 13, 14
Points 10 and 11 are right below the occipital bone,
1 to 2 inches from the center of the spine. Point 12 is
underneath C7, the seventh cervical vertebrae. Points 13
and 14 are 1 to 2 inches away from Point 12. Point 1 is
over the thyroid gland.

Zone 2
Area of the lower back
Points 15, 16, 17
Point 15 is located on L2-3, between the second and
third lumbar vertebrae. Points 16 and 17 are on the same
level as Point 15 and are at 1 to 2 inch intervals.

Zone 3
Area of the liver
Points 3, 4, 5, 6
Points 4, 5, and 6 are right below the right bottom
rib. Point 3 is located on the bottom tip of the xiphoid
process, which is the bottom part of the sternum.

Zone 4
Area of the stomach
Points 7, 8, 9
Points 7, 8 and 9 are 1 to 2 inches away from the
belly button.

Zone 5
Area of the chest
Point 2
Point 2 is located down the middle on the same level
as the fifth rib.

Procedure Overview:

Sessions are conducted 1 to 2 times a week. The
condition of the patient and the specific type of allergy
both help to determine the treatment zones. Treatments
are especially effective when an allergy causes a
disturbance in microcirculation and lymphatic ability to
function. Points 1, 2, 10, 11, 12, 13, and 14 may be used
in any course of treatment against allergies.

Quantity of attachments:

2 to 3 per session during a strong allergic reaction
5 to 6 per session during a remission or a weaker
reaction

Quantity of sessions:

Use 6 to 8 sessions with about 2 to 3 courses of healing.

Combination healing:

Leech therapy provides supplementary support during
allergy treatment. Its main purpose is to restore the
vein and lymphatic systems. A lot of people forgo the
possibility of healing without taking medication, but
there are great methods out there: cleansing the skin,
stomach, and liver, breathing exercises, medicinal herbs.
Proper fasting techniques are also very effective.

Leech therapy and surgery

Leech therapy is very effective during many postoperative
complications: pneumonia, slow healing of wounds, formation
of scar tissues, and abnormal connections between two organs or
vessels that normally do not connect (*fistulas*). The principals of
this healing process with leech therapy are similar to the ones of
chronic bronchitis or a non-healing wound (see those sections).

Leech therapy has also been very effective following heart
surgery. Its main focus has been the prevention of complications
involving thrombosis and blood clots in the heart. It has been
shown to be extremely effective in these cases, but it must be
administered with the supervision of an experienced doctor
who can closely monitor the procedure. *(Note: This procedure will
be outlined in more detail in the next edition when there is enough
clinical evidence to provide real testimony of success.)*

Inflammatory skin and hypodermic diseases

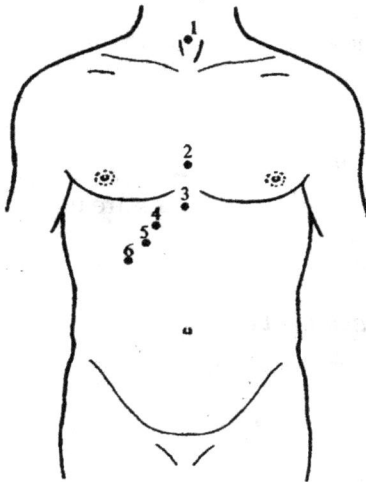

A trauma, puncture, or splinter can become an immediate cause of these diseases. Oftentimes, they lead to a weakened immune function and result in the skin's inability to defend and heal itself. It should be noted, however, that leech therapy can only be used on the affected area when a complication is in its initial stage. Otherwise, it is used to stimulate the immune system and help regulate healthy blood circulation. When suffering from boils, only a specialist should administer leech therapy since it has a higher chance of complications.

Attachment Zones:

Zone 1
Points on the affected area or nearby

Zone 2
Area of the liver
Points 3, 4, 5, and 6
Points 4, 5, and 6 are right below the right bottom
rib. Point 3 is located on the bottom tip of the xiphoid
process, which is the bottom part of the sternum.

Zone 3
Area of the chest
Point 2
Point 2 is in the middle and on the same level as the fifth rib.

Procedure Overview:

During procedures all the zones are used in combination.

Quantity of attachments:

1 to 4 per session depending on the size of the area affected.

Quantity of sessions:

Administer 4 to 5 sessions every other day. The course of healing is 10 to 12 sessions altogether depending on the condition. Course of healing may be repeated if needed.

Combination healing:

Leech therapy is done alongside a cleansing of the organism. Helpful cleansers include wheat sprouts, mumijo, and cleansing teas.

Varicose veins

This is a disease connected with a weakening structure of the veins' walls that causes them to stretch and swell. Although varicose veins are easily noticeable, as a rule, it is a sign that the entire circulatory system is suffering to some extent. Depending on the person's lifestyle and type of work, the disease can manifest itself in different places of the body but the legs are affected most often.

People who suffer from varicose veins are usually the ones who are engaged in rigorous physical work or who are on their feet a lot. The consequences of this condition can affect the whole body, even if to a minor extent, and may lead to headaches, constipation, liver problems and gall bladder problems. Some women may even face chronic diseases of the reproductive system.

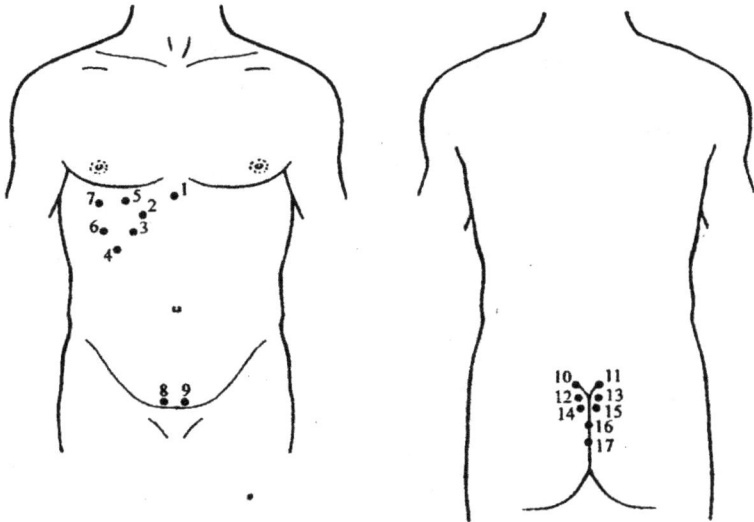

Attachment Zones:

Zone 1
Area of the tailbone
Points 10-15, 16, 17
Points 16 and 17 are located on the bottom tip of the tailbone. Points 10-15 are outlining the sacrum.

Zone 2
Area of the pubic bone
Points 8 and 9
Points 8 and 9 are placed over the pubic bone

Zone 3
Area of the liver

Points 1-7
Points 2, 3 and 4 are right underneath the right bottom rib. Points 5, 6 and 7 are over the liver. Point 1 is located on the tip of the xiphoid process, which is the bottom part of the sternum.

Zone 4
The affected area
Points 1-12
Points 1-7 are positioned in a checkered manner alongside the varicose vein. And Points 8-12 are also placed in a similar style around the skin of brownish pigmentation near the tip of the extremity.

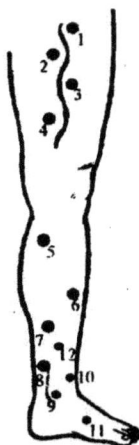

Procedure Overview:

Combine Zones 1-3 with the affected area zone.

Quantity of attachments:

Quantity is closely related to the condition of the veins. As a general rule, two attachments from Zone 1 or 2 are combined with 3 to 4 attachments alongside the vein.

Quantity of sessions:

Administer twice a week when there are no signs of inflammation. Course of healing is 9-11 sessions.

Combination healing:

Leech therapy may be combined with breathing exercises and exercises designed for varicose illnesses.

Acute and chronic thrombophlebitis (*blood clots*)

Thrombophlebitis is caused by blood clots blocking a regular blood flow through veins. It is frequently accompanied by hypostasis and pain. The suffering person may by bedridden for 3 to 4 weeks at a time. Quite often, acute thrombophlebitis develops into a chronic condition. There is hardly a better approach to this type of varicose disease than a timely application of a medicinal leech. If leeches are applied in the early stages, when only a reddening of the veins (*phlebitis*) is detected, then it is possible to prevent the development of blood clots.

Attachment Zones:

Treatment is administered on the border of the affected reddening area, alongside the vein.
(Note: See the zones and diagrams from the varicose vein section to use during treatments.)

Procedure Overview:

Never place a leech directly on a vein.

Quantity of attachments:

3 to 8 per session depending on the condition of the disease

Quantity of sessions:

During acute stages, sessions are held daily until the pain goes away. Then they are held 2 to 3 times a week until all signs of the disease are gone. Zones 2 and 3 (from the varicose section) are only used after the redness is gone. The healing course may be repeated after two months.

Combination healing:

Leech therapy can be the primary, and the most effective, choice of treatment. Only when the sharp pain is alleviated, the patient may use additional treatment methods such as the ones listed in the varicose vein section.

Non-healing wounds

Most often, non-healing wounds are the results of circulatory problems and blood clots, and lead to the tissue's inability to heal. Leeches can improve microcirculation, blood circulation, while removing hypostasis, blood stasis, and stimulating the immune system, which helps to clean and heal the wound.

Attachment Zones:

Zone 1
Around and on the affected area.

Zone 2
Points alongside swollen veins (similar to the style shown in the varicose vein section)

Other Zones
Also areas of the liver, pubic bone, and tailbone (the same ones shown in the varicose vein section)

Procedure Overview:

During the course of healing, points on the affected area are combined with points in alternating Zones 2, 3, and 4. When faced with a trophic ulcer, do not place a leech on the edge of a wound but rather about 1 to 2 inches away. For the most part, though, leeches are placed right on the wound (even though it is difficult to do at times because the fluids excreted by the wound repulse them). *(Note: Placing a leech on the wound may generate incredible healing results.)*

Quantity of attachments:

3 to 8 per session depending on the size of the wound

Quantity of sessions:

The schedule is designed based on the condition of the wound. At first, sessions can be held daily until the wound is clean. Then, they can be continued every other day, and then as needed. For the most part, 3 to 4 sessions are sufficient to start the healing process. In the most extreme cases, however, 15 to 20 sessions may be required, alongside other methods of cleansing the wound and stimulating the immune system.

Combination healing:

Leech therapy is an effective means of treatment; however, keep in mind that chronic wounds may be the result of the body's deteriorated metabolism. If this is the case, then it becomes necessary to cleanse the liver, cleanse the colon, and engage in breathing exercises. Also, the wound may be treated externally with natural remedies—herbs, cabbage leaves, aloe, silver water, etc.

Acute and chronic hemorrhoids and fissures

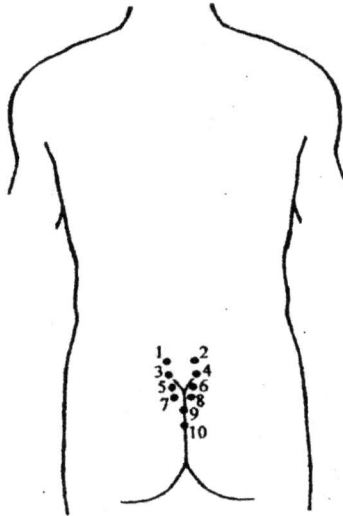

As a general rule, hemorrhoids develop when there are complications in the veins. Quite often, external hemorrhoids develop into thrombosis (*formation of a blood clot*). Using compresses, lotions, and hemorrhoid suppositories are ineffective in treating the root of the problem. It is necessary to combine holistic and local points of attachment to reduce blood stasis. Leech therapy can produce great results.

Attachment Zones:

Zone 1
Area around the anus and the hemorrhoids

Zone 2
Area around the tailbone
Points 1-10
Points 9 and 10 are located on the bottom tip of the tailbone. Points 1-8 are outlining the sacrum.

Procedure Overview:

During acute hemorrhoids or a sudden inflammation, the leech is placed right on the knot, which leads to a drastic reduction in pain and the diffusion of the blood clot.

Quantity of attachments:

2 to 3 per session (leave the leeches on until they fall off on their own)

Quantity of sessions:

Daily until the pain goes away.

Combination healing:

After leech therapy is used to relieve the knots, supplemental methods may be used to reduce the blood in the area of the anal canal. Physical exercise, massage, intestinal cleansing, liver cleansing, and any action against constipation (i.e. increasing fiber) are all good options in this case.

Mastitis and galactostasis

The development of galactostasis is connected with disruption of milk outflow, its stagnation, and the infection that follows. Mastitis is the inflammation of the mammary gland. Using leech therapy is a great treatment during initial stages when the pain just starts and the redness becomes visible on the mammary gland.

Attachment Zones:

Zone1
The affected area: the lump and the skin showing redness (Points 5, 6, and 7)

Zone 2
Area of the sternum
Points 1-4 are located on the sternum between the
third and fifth rib

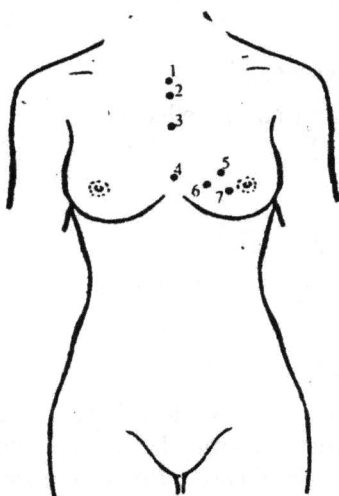

Procedure Overview:

Sessions are administered until the problem starts
reversing itself—less pain, less redness, and a
reduction in swelling.

Quantity of attachments:

3 to 4 per session

Quantity of sessions:

Sessions are held daily until the pain decreases.
Then, sessions are conducted every other day until
the healing process is complete.

Combination healing:

If leech therapy is used early enough, then it
may be the only treatment required.

Bone fracture and infection of the bone (*osteomyelitis*)

Often after the cast is removed, there is a range of problems:
poor circulation in the area, lack of elasticity in the joints, muscle
weakness, and a lagging bone callus replacement. In all these
cases, and especially when dealing with open fractures, leech
therapy can enhance the healing process.

Attachment Zones:

During fractures and bone infections, leech therapy
should only be used on the affected area such as the
fractured bone, the nearby joint, and the area
of the affected bone.

Procedure Overview:

Sessions are held until full recovery.

Quantity of attachments:

3 to 5 per session

Quantity of sessions:

2 to 3 sessions are conducted per week. Course of
healing usually includes 9 to 15 sessions.

Combination healing:

Leech therapy should be used alongside physical
therapy, massage, herbal medicine, mumijo (during
open fractures), and also stimulants of the immune
system when there is a bone infection.

Radiculitis

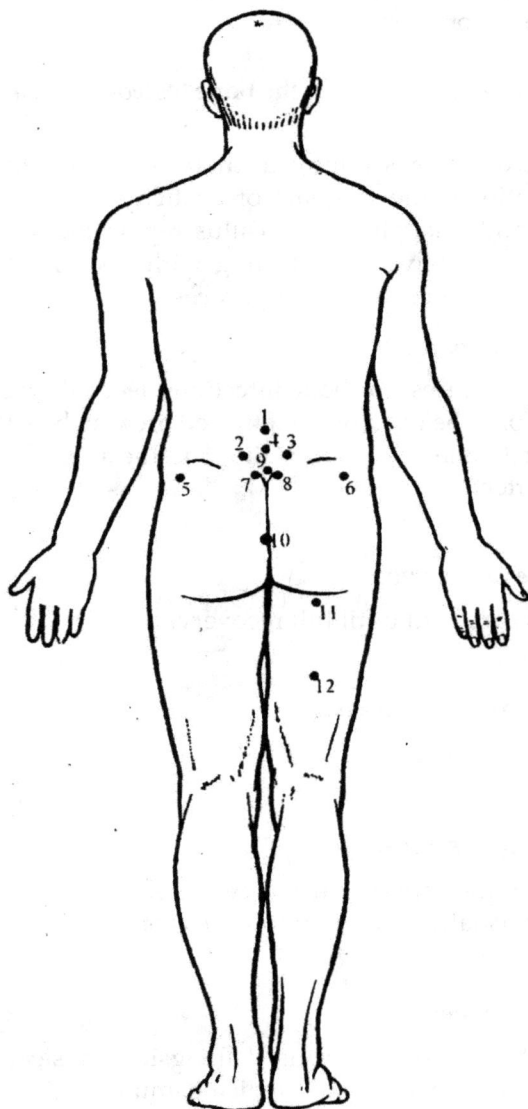

Radicular pain is a pain shooting out from the nerve root, which is connected to the spine. In some instances, this pain stems from internal swelling and blood stasis in the spinal area. Usually, the skin of the affected area becomes puffy. The pain becomes more intense while resting and subsides during physical movement. In these cases, leech therapy can provide healing support.

Attachment Zones:

Zone 1
Points 1, 2, 3, 4
The affected area: the area that has the most pain
(Points 1-4).

Zone 2
Area around the tailbone
Points 7, 8, 9 and 10
Point 10 is located on the bottom tip of the tailbone.
Points 7, 8 and 9 are outlining the sacrum.

Zone 3
Area of the buttocks
Points 5 and 6 are placed on the most painful points
on the buttocks.

Zone 4
Affected area that goes along the sciatic nerve
Points 11 and 12 are placed along the sciatic nerve.

Procedure Overview:

If there is no improvement after the third session, then leech therapy is not the right course of treatment.

Quantity of attachments:

5 to 6 per session

Quantity of sessions:

The first 3 to 4 sessions are held daily until the pain subsides. The entire course of healing is 8 to 10 sessions.

Combination healing:

When radicular pain is accompanied by internal inflammation, poor blood circulation and venous stasis, leech therapy should be combined with physical therapy.

Bruises and traumas

Any trauma is accompanied by tissue damage, swelling, capillary injury, and formation of hematomas. Quite often traumas can lead to other serious conditions: retinal detachment, worsened eyesight, thrombophlebitis (blood clots), post traumatic inflammation, arachnoiditis, arthritis, etc. Leech therapy is able to provide indispensible help in these cases.

Attachment Zones:

The affected area

Procedure Overview:

Leech therapy may be used the same day that the trauma occurs. This helps prevent further complications.

Quantity of attachments:

3 to 4 per session

Quantity of sessions:

The first 2 to 3 sessions are conducted daily; then, 2 to 3 times per week. The length of the healing course depends on the degree of the trauma and the complications that may arise because of it.

Combination healing:

Leech therapy should be used in combination with physical therapy and massage.

Gynecology

During treatment of gynecologic diseases, leeches can be used not only on the surface but also internally. When leeches are placed on the right or left vaginal walls, those sessions should only be conducted under the supervision of a gynecologist.

Leeches can be very effective in helping against inflammation of the uterus and fallopian tubes. During leech therapy, the hormonal balance is restored quicker allowing the entire organism to recover faster. Furthermore, some other general diseases occur simultaneously with sexual hormone disorders. In these cases, it is recommended to use leeches internally as well.

(It should be noted, however, that there are not many experts in the United States to apply the methods described for the diseases of the female reproductive system.)

Kidney diseases

Leech therapy is a good treatment in combination with other methods during kidney problems, such as glomerulonephritis *(damaged kidney filtration system, which helps clean the blood from waste)*, kidney failure and kidney damage from trauma.

Attachment Zones:

Zone 1
Area of the lower back
Points 1-11
Point 1 is located at L2-3, second or third lumbar vertebrae. Points 2, 3, 6, 7, 8 and 9 are spaced from the center point at 1 to 2 inch intervals. Points 4 and 5, 10 and 11 are above and below Points 2 and 3, respectively. In addition, other points may be used in the area especially those that are painful to touch.

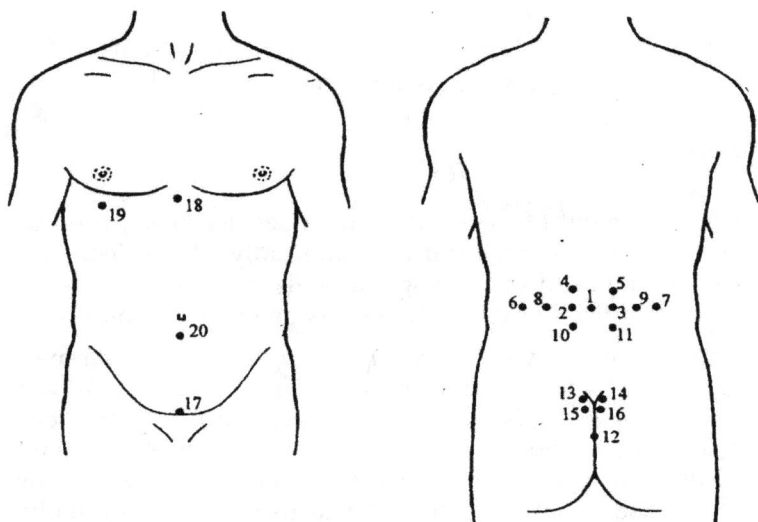

Zone 2
Area of the tailbone
Points 12, 13, 14, 15, 16
Point 12 is located on the bottom tip of the tailbone.
Points 13-16 are outlining the sacrum.

Zone 3
Area of the lower stomach
Points 17 and 20
Point 20 is 2 to 3 inches below the belly button. Point 17
is over the pubic bone.

Zone 4
Area of the liver
Points 18 and 19
Point 18 is located on the tip of the xiphoid process,
which is the bottom part of the sternum. Point 19 is
underneath the sixth rib.

Procedure Overview:

The lower back area is the main target area for the
treatment. When treating glomerulonephritis, the points

over the thyroid gland and the sternum are included as well. When treating kidney failure, the area of the liver becomes very important. And points near the tailbone become particularly important when there are signs of hyperemia *(excess of blood)* in the intestinal area.

Quantity of attachments:

2 to 3 per session during glomerulonephritis
7 to 8 per session during trauma and treatment of nephritic insufficiency (in the absence of anaemia)

Quantity of sessions:

First 5 to 7 sessions are held every other day and then, twice a week. Course of healing is 7 to 12 sessions. Usually the course needs to be repeated.

Combination healing:

During glomerulonephritis, leech therapy is conducted only under the supervision of a doctor who is constantly monitoring the results and the immune system. When done incorrectly, the condition may worsen. With glomerulonephritis or kidney failure, it is absolutely necessary to use other methods such as medicinal herbs and cleansing processes, while working to activate the lungs as well. Unfortunately, only a few very experienced specialists have the ability to effectively cure these two diseases.

Prostate

Adenoma (*a benign tumor*) and inflammation of the prostate gland (*chronic prostatitis*) usually result from venous stasis in the area (and at times after gonorrhea). During prostatitis, an infection occurs while adenoma is accompanied by an enlarged prostate which may interfere with the urination process. In either case, sexual functions are affected. By restoring the proper blood circulation in the area, leech therapy attacks the core of the disease, thus making it a good treatment in combination with other methods.

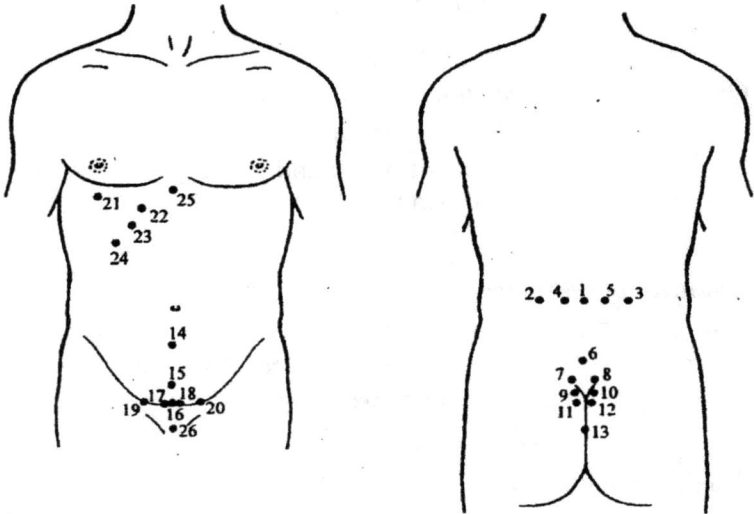

Attachment Zones:

Zone 1
Area of the pubic bone
Points 16, 17, 18, 26
Point 16 is over the pubic bone. Points 17 and 18 are a half an inch away from Point 16. Point 26 is right over the sex organ.

Zone 2
Area of the lower stomach
Points 14, 15, 19, 20
Point 15 is 2 to 3 inches above Point 16. Point 14 is 2 to 3 inches below the belly button. Points 19 and 20 are in the area of the groin.

Zone 3
Area of the tailbone
Points 6-13

Point 13 is located on the bottom tip of the tailbone.
Points 6-12 are outlining the sacrum.

Zone 4
Lower back area
Points 1-5
Point 1 is located at L2-3, second or third lumbar
vertebrae. Points 2-5 are spaced from the center
point at 1 to 2 inch intervals.

Zone 5
Area of the liver
Points 21, 22, 23, 24, 25
Points 22, 23, and 24 are right underneath the right
bottom rib. Point 21 is over the area of the liver. Point 25
is located on the tip of the xiphoid process, which is the
bottom part of the sternum.

Procedure Overview:

Sessions are conducted with more attention on Zones
1, 2, and 3. Zones 4 and 5 are not used more than once
during a course of treatment and, as a general rule, they
are used at the end. The most important points are over
the affected area. This treatment should be administered
under the supervision of an urologist.

Quantity of attachment:

3 to 5 per session

Quantity of sessions:

Sessions are held every other day. Course of healing
is 12 sessions. Usually it takes 3 to 4 courses for a
complete healing, although there should be tremendous
improvement after just the first course.

Combination healing:

It is necessary to use leech therapy along with physical exercises, breathing exercises, and other methods of increasing the metabolism.

Glaucoma

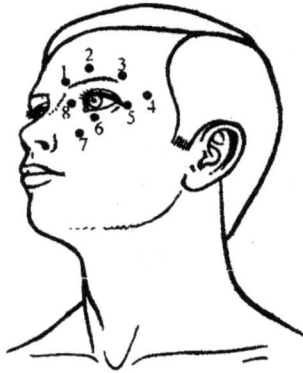

Glaucoma is usually accompanied by a constant or periodic increase of intraocular pressure and nerve damage in the eye. The cause is usually rooted in poorly functioning fluid regulation in the eye, which suffers when the amount of fluid increases along with the pressure.

Leech therapy acts as a great defense against primary causes of this disease. During a period of increased pressure, leech therapy works quickly, within thirty to forty-five minutes. *(Note: This method may be used to treat the underlying disease or a just a flare up in pressure. Either way, leech therapy improves fluids circulation while reducing the swelling, and ridding the organism of vascular diseases.)*

Attachment Zones:

Zone 1
Area around the eye
Points 1, 2, 3, 4, 5, 6, 7, 8
Points 5 and 8 are positioned just outside the corners of the eye. Points 1, 2, 3 are positioned slightly over the eyebrow on both sides and the middle. Point 4

is positioned over the temple. Point 6 is underneath the eye. Point 7 is positioned about half an inch below Point 6.

Zone 2
Back of the neck area (similar to the zones used for allergies)
Points are placed right below the occipital bone, 1 to 2 inches from the center of the spine.

Zone 3
Area of the liver
Points are placed right below the right bottom rib and over the liver. One point is located on the tip of the xiphoid process, which is the bottom part of the sternum.

Procedure Overview:

During course of treatment, leeches are first placed in Zone 1, and left on until they fall off on their own. After 3 to 4 sessions, points from Zones 2 and 3 are used as well.

Quantity of attachments:

2 to 3 per session

Quantity of sessions:

Course of healing is 11 sessions. It should be repeated once or twice with 1 to 2 month intervals in between. The frequency and intensity should depend on the intraocular pressure.

Combination healing:

To reach maximum effectiveness, use hydrotherapy as well.

Inflammatory diseases of the eye

This includes numerous diseases: keratitis, iridocyclitis, uveitis, chorioretinitis, etc. The causing source may be infection, trauma, poor blood circulation, etc. Leeches ultimately provide the necessary help when faced with these diseases because they possess anti-inflammatory substances, which have the ability to reduce swelling and promote healthy lymphatic processes. Leech therapy can also prevent complications, which are frequent during these types of diseases.

Attachment Zones:

The same ones as in the glaucoma section.

Procedure Overview:

Usually leeches are attached to the affected side. During course of treatment, leeches are first placed on two or three points, until they fall off on their own, in Zone 1. After 3 to 4 sessions, start including points in Zones 2. After three more sessions, start using points in Zone 3.

Quantity of attachments:

2 to 3 per session

Quantity of sessions:

The length of the course of treatment is determined by the severity of the condition as well as the reaction to the treatment. If it is absolutely necessary, the course may be repeated, but usually even the first few sessions provide a substantial relief.

Combination healing:

You may add compresses with medicinal herbs to the treatment as well as silver water.

Other diseases of the eye

There are numerous other eye diseases. Because of their rarity, however, there is not enough clinical practice to supply evidence of success with leech therapy. Based on the above examples though, leech therapy may soon prove to be useful in healing these diseases as well. Leech therapy can be especially important during severe complications, such as a sympathetic inflammation (*when both eyes experience complications after only one suffers the trauma*), and also during progression of retinal detachment, provided that a patient is trained properly to conduct the procedure at home or a doctor with experience helps administer it.

Stuffy nose from allergies or a sinus infection

A stuffy nose is most often caused by a chronic or acute inflammation in the nose due to a number of causes: viruses, bacteria, air pollution or other irritants. Sinusitis is an inflammation of the sinuses, which is caused by internal reactions like an infection, allergy, or autoimmune issue. Leech therapy is especially effective when the mucous membrane becomes swollen. It is also effective for treating an abnormal growth on the mucous membrane of the nose (*a polyp*), which may develop during bouts of hay fever and inflammation of the nasal passages.

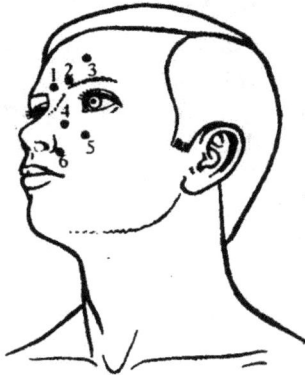

Attachment Zones:

Zone 1
Middle of the face area
Points 1-6
Points 4 and 6 are located on the edge of the nose. Points 1, 2, 3, and 5 are located over the paranasal sinuses.

Zone 2
Internal area of the nose
Points are placed along the lower third of the septum.

Procedure Overview:

Usually sessions include points that are symmetrically located. *(Note: Attachments along the septum should only be made by a specialist.)*

Quantity of attachments:

2 to 3 per session

Quantity of sessions:

If a stuffy nose is accompanied by blood stasis, then breathing improves tremendously just after one leech therapy session. Sessions are held with 2 to 3 day breaks in between. Course of healing is usually 5 to 7 sessions. When treating hay fever, it is also important to include the zones shown in the allergies section.

Combination healing:

Leech therapy may be combined with breathing exercises.

Ear diseases

Leech therapy provides help in such cases as acoustic neuroma, Ménière's disease, labyrinthitis (*an inflammation of the inner ear*), acute and chronic otitis (*ear inflammations*), and ear trauma.

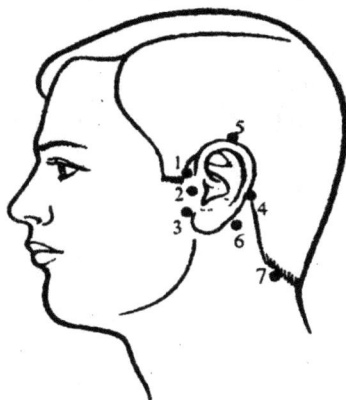

Attachment Zones:

Zone 1
Area around the ear
Points 1-5
Points 1-5 are placed around the ear.

Zone 2
Back of the neck area
Point 6 is right over the mastoid process. Point 7 is right below the occipital bone and 2 to 3 inches from the spine.

Procedure Overview:

Leeches are placed until they fall off on their own.

Quantity of attachments:

2 to 3 per session

Quantity of sessions:

8 to 10 sessions are held per course. Usually 2 to 3 courses are required. During chronic diseases, sessions are held twice a week. For Ménière's disease or acoustic neuroma, leech therapy courses should be repeated.

Combination healing:

Leech therapy may be combined with acupuncture.

8

Leech Therapy at Home

Choosing leech therapy

By now, you are already familiar with the great gifts that nature has bestowed upon this little worm. And you are probably wondering whether it is possible to use leech therapy at home safely and effectively to heal yourself. A simple answer is—yes. The more precise answer is that by combining your specialist's expertise and the information from this book you should be able to recognize if your situation requires the help of a leech and how to use it to your maximum benefit.

It is important to reiterate that leech therapy will only lead to significant results if used properly and under the right circumstances. Certainly, it would be unrealistic to begin looking at medicinal leeches as the next panacea—a remedy for all diseases. These unrealistic expectations and magical thinking may have formed after reading previous chapters that describe so many cases of leech therapy applications, such as heart problems, liver diseases, allergies, etc. Yet, you must remember that leech therapy does not target any one single organ in the body, but is an effective and natural way to improve blood circulation in the area of the attachment and thus helps the entire organism in the healing process. And in certain conditions, the application of medicinal leeches treats the core causes of a disease by diffusing the stasis of blood and fluids in veins and tissues, which suffer from blockages and a deteriorating metabolism.

You can expect to achieve great results with leech therapy only if the instructions are scrupulously followed. It should be emphasized, however, that the general understanding of leech therapy is that, while we put ourselves in the hands of doctors and nature to treat us, we are ultimately responsible for our health.

Ten rules of leech therapy

Rule #1: Identify the problem.

It is usually the best, if the specialist has particularly advised—or advised against—the use of leeches in your case. Therefore, before making a final determination, consult with a specialist to make sure you understand the reasons for the worsening of your health condition and the core causes of your disease, such as:
- Venous stasis, high blood pressure
- Tissue swelling
- Inflammatory process
- Deterioration of microcirculation and damaged metabolism, atrophy
- Immune deficiency

Rule #2: Do no harm.

Revisit the earlier chapters and review all the factors that could yield negative outcomes. *(Note: It is very important to maintain a safe amount of hemoglobin in the blood throughout the course of treatment. This may be achieved by eating food rich in iron.)*

Rule #3: Having the right map is the key to success.

Almost any specialist can refer to the diagrams in this book to identify necessary points of attachment for a particular disease. However, it is highly recommended to consult with a specialist about what specific zones and points are right for you.

Rule #4: A knowledgeable doctor/specialist is the best assistant.

It is important to reach a full understanding of the process from start to finish before proceeding on your own. Therefore, conduct the initial procedures with a specialist at your side before attempting any self-treatment. This should eliminate any fears, help you gain confidence, and provide you with the right knowledge to work safely and comfortably with leeches and open wounds.

Rule #5: The road to health begins with a healthy leech.

It is imperative that you only use leeches from a trusted source where they have been grown in an artificial environment. These places quarantine their leeches, breed them in controlled environments, and certify that the leeches have been properly prepared. (*Note: Leeches can get sick too. Do not use leeches caught in the wild or buy any homegrown leeches from an unknown source. You should always purchase leeches from a reputable and reliable place.*)

Rule #6: Keep all necessities handy.

Sessions will go more smoothly when proper preparations are made, and all the steps are carefully demonstrated by a specialist during the first few sessions. Before you begin a session make sure to prepare, and keep within your reach, the following items:
- Narrow and wide sterile bandages;
- Cotton balls;
- Hydrogen peroxide, iodine, rubbing alcohol, and thrombin powder, which may be used to stop strong bleeding;

- Cold water and ice (although ice is seldom used);
- Clean sheets, large and small (to prevent staining clothes with blood).

Rule #7: Do not put it where it should not be.

Leech therapy can only help when applied to the right spot at the right time. Follow the specialist's instructions; and do not proceed until you are absolutely sure that you understand the procedure. If in doubt, seek help immediately! When conducting a session at home on your own, do not place leeches on the following spots:

- Mucous membranes (tongue, gums, vagina, inside a nose);
- Directly over veins;
- On the neck and/or mammary glands.

Rule #8: Attachment is the key to a successful treatment.

Leech therapy is beneficial only when a leech is properly attached. Usually, the attachment process does not pose any complex problems. A thorough review of the previous chapters is indispensible; but here is a brief summary of the process:

- Before attempting the attachment, prepare the skin properly (preferably leaving the skin clean and without any smells).
- Put a leech in a small glass or tube and place it over the point on the body you wish the leech to attach to. Leave it on until the leech attaches. If this does not happen within 3 to 4 minutes, use other methods described earlier in the book.
- After the leech breaks through the skin, there might be either a slight sting; or you may feel no pain at all. Then the leech will make itself more comfortable by attaching with the bottom sucker as well and begin sucking the blood.

- Observe the leech. At first, the sucking motion is subtle and very difficult to notice. But over time, as the leech delves deeper into the tissue and takes up more territory on the skin, it becomes easier for the leech to suck blood. At this point, it begins to suck faster, and you will notice the increased sucking motion, as well as its growth in size. *(Note: This is the exact moment when the leech is removed if it needs to be detached manually, as discussed in earlier chapters. In this case, the leech will still benefit the organism, but with a limited loss of blood.)*

Rule #9: If you need to stop, then stop.

Do not hesitate to stop the procedure if you absolutely have to. In case of an unscheduled removal of the leech, you may put a pinch of salt on its back or gently wipe it down with iodine. However, in most cases, the leech is left on until it falls off on its own.

Rule #10: A strong finish is more important that strong start.

Following a session, treating the wound, bandaging, and taking care of the bleeding are all important aspects of leech therapy. Some people become tense or uncomfortable when bleeding continues after the leech's detachment. But, it is important to remember that bleeding following a session is absolutely normal and, in most cases, extremely healthy. Usually, about 20 to 30 ml of blood will exit the wound per attachment, although it is not unusual for the wound to bleed for up to twenty-four hours.

After the leech falls off, the wound is treated with gauze. Then, for the first 2 to 3 hours, wrap it tightly, but not so that you are cutting off the blood flow in the veins. Use your common sense here. If blood seeps through the bandage, do not remove it but, instead, add another layer on top of it. In rare cases, if the bandage becomes entirely soaked with blood, you may remove the bandage, treat the wound with hydrogen peroxide, and re-bandage tightly with a new gauze. You may also place a bag of ice over the bandage to speed up the process.

Depending on the condition, replace the bandage in six, twelve, or twenty-four hour intervals. Observe the wound. Most often, it will have already stopped bleeding. Make sure to write down the time and let your specialist know how long the wound was bleeding—it may have significant diagnostic implications.

Shared responsibilities

The process of healing and leech therapy requires active participation by all three parties: the patient, the specialist, and the leech. Although the roles and responsibilities of each are different, they all share the common goal in the healing process. By recognizing these shared goals and responsibilities we can take the safest and most effective steps towards our recovery.

The specialist:

The specialist, or attending physician, should:
- Prepare all necessities for the procedure;
- Choose healthy leeches;
- Create a comfortable and relaxed atmosphere;
- Attach leeches and treat the wounds after they fall off;
- Decide how long the wound should bleed afterwards;
- Know how to care for fresh and used leeches;
- Understand how to squeeze out the blood from the full leech;
- Teach the entire process (from start to finish) to a patient.

The saying goes, "give a man a fish and you will feed him for a day, but teach him how to fish, and you will feed him for a lifetime." This is the approach that doctors should have with their patients. It is the responsibility of a doctor to teach a patient how to "fish" for health.

The patient:

The patient should diligently follow directions while working towards a healthy body and mind.

The leech:

Being one of the few true natural ways for a person to regain a healthy life, the leech begins to help its patient within the first minutes of contact. Nature gave leeches the ability to heal; but to achieve necessary results one should make sure that leeches being used are healthy and live in an environment that mirrors their natural surroundings (whether they are in a lab or at home).

9

Final Thoughts

If the current trend continues, we may soon see the medicinal leech reclaim its rightful place in standard medicinal practices. Recently this belief has taken a strong hold among users; and it stems from many possible applications this wonderful little creature has in dermatology, neuropathology, oncology, ophthalmology, stomatology, therapy, surgery, obstetrics, and gynecology, just to name a few.

While the effects of leech therapy are similar to that of pharmaceutical drugs, it has obvious and invaluable advantages. For once, leeches are natural healers. In addition, unlike pills, leech therapy is not accompanied by a wide array of side effects. Moreover, leeches affect the entire organism to help it to repair several damaged organs simultaneously. All the while, the application of leeches can be conducted in hospitals, doctors' offices, and even at home.

Finally, it works fast. The quick-acting leech not only reduces the patient's suffering but also allows both, the patient and the doctor, to assess the effectiveness of the procedure promptly —a benefit that pills oftentimes do not offer for weeks or even months.

It has to be emphasized, though, that leeches will not help a person who is psychologically set against them—usually, they will not even attach. Therefore, not only the specialists but the person being treated should feel positively about these little healers and be thankful for their work.

Although it is highly unlikely that a doctor, who has been taught by our universities' standard practice of medicine, would agree to use leeches as the sole treatment for an illness, this is another matter altogether when we come across a healer who uses traditional medicine. In the best of both worlds scenario, a doctor and a leech therapist, who have a vast amount of experience with natural remedies, would choose to work together to offer a patient the best chance for a recovery. Ideally, a possible equation should look like this:

DOCTOR + PATIENT + LEECH SPECIALIST + LEECH = HEALING PROCESS.

It is then that leech therapy will become both a science and an art.

Of course, this process will take time to develop, for it is not the usual style of modern medicine, where people are forced into the "here, take this pill three times a day and come back in a month" system. In leech therapy, each individual is required to be treated as one, with constant supervision and a tailored treatment to each particular person and circumstance. Consequently, everyone (specialist and patient, maybe even family) involved in leech therapy would need to talk through their responsibilities and understand the entire process.

Certainly, the procedure of leech therapy is quite unusual—in fact, it is a mini-surgical procedure that requires patience, time and effort—but just like with anything else, what you get out of it is what you put into it.

Remember, leech therapy is not simply a mechanical process of bleeding, or just an exchange of money between the doctor and the patient, but a complex journey to healing that requires constant attention from the doctor and a shared responsibility by the patient. Only if it is correctly applied by educated specialists and users, it will become possible for us to further unlock the powers of this wonderful treatment.

10

<u>Appendix</u>

Mapping your healing points

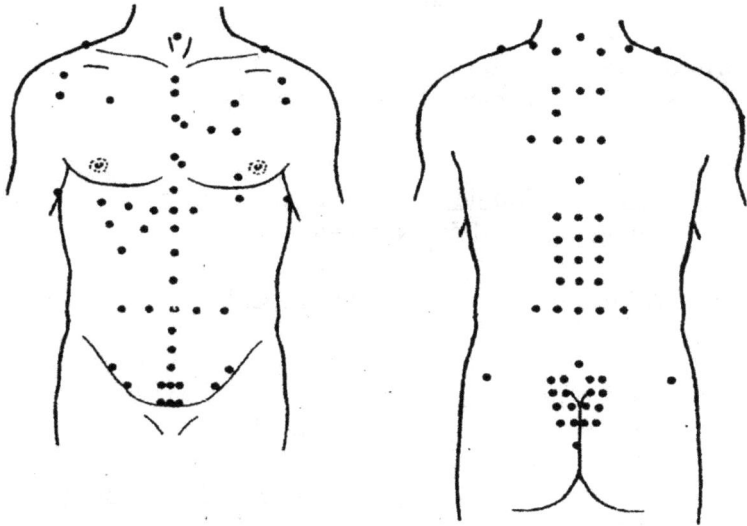

Bibliography

Cavinov, Vladimir and Tatiana Pavlova. Leech: the healer of all. Moscow: Dealya, 2007.

Garashenko, Larissa. Healing With Leeches In Household Conditions. Moscow: ACT-Press, 2007.

Garashenko, Larissa, and Genadi Nekonoff. Leech Therapy Can Help You: The Hirudotherapy Encyclopedia. Moscow: Astrel, 2005.

"Hirudotherapy." Med-Center April 15, 2011 <http://www.mederbis.com.ua/node/90>

"Hirudotherapy: Method of Healing." Eurasia the Clinic of Western Medicine. April 10, 2011 <http://www.ru03. ru/index.php?Main_Name=metod_gerudo>

Kamenev, Yurii, and Oleg Kamenev. A leech can help you. Ves, 2009.

Kazmin, Victor. Leeches are for your health. Simple. Effective. Safe. Barrow Press, 2005.

Stoyanovskiy, Daniel. Medicinal Leech and Blood Letting. Stalkerr, 2009.

About the Author

Born and raised in Soviet Russia, Matt Isaac emigrated
from St. Petersburg, Russia to Cleveland, Ohio shortly after
the collapse of the Berlin Wall. Ever since his immigration,
he found himself fascinated with the different approaches
to medicine between his old country and new; so after years
of investigation, he decided to write his first book on leech
therapy—a therapy that is highly accepted and respected
in one country, and completely humored
and ignored in the other.

Leech Therapy

ORDER FORM

Additional copies of **Leech Therapy: An Introduction to a Natural Healing Alternative** may be purchased through most online retailers or ordered through your local bookstore.

To obtain copies directly from the publisher, you may mail a check or money order payable to:

HEALTH BY PROFESSION
P O Box 24775
Cleveland, OH 44124

Please send _____ (number of) copies of **Leech Therapy** to:

Name: _____

Company:_____

Address: _____

City, State, Zip: _____

Telephone: _____ Email: _____

Quantity: Price per book:

1	$19.95
2-9	$17.95
10-49	$15.95
50+	Please contact us for special pricing

Pricing includes shipping within 48 contiguous United States. Please contact us to determine costs elsewhere.

Questions? Contact us at:
www.LeechTherapy.info

www.ingramcontent.com/pod-product-compliance
Lightning Source LLC
Chambersburg PA
CBHW070250290326
41930CB00041B/2430